# Let's Walk Through

."From the heart & mind
to paper to person to profession"

## Aditi Tathagat Gosalia

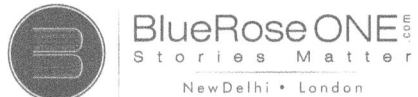

**BLUEROSE PUBLISHERS**
India | U.K.

Copyright © Aditi Tathagat Gosalia 2024

All rights reserved by author. No part of this publication may be reproduced, stored in a retrieval system, or transmitted in any form or by any means, electronic, mechanical, photocopying, recording or otherwise, without the prior permission of the author. Although every precaution has been taken to verify the accuracy of the information contained herein, the publisher assumes no responsibility for any errors or omissions. No liability is assumed for damages that may result from the use of information contained within.

BlueRose Publishers takes no responsibility for any damages, losses, or liabilities that may arise from the use or misuse of the information, products, or services provided in this publication.

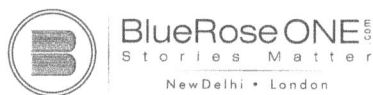

For permissions requests or inquiries regarding this publication, please contact:

BLUEROSE PUBLISHERS
www.BlueRoseONE.com
info@bluerosepublishers.com
+91 8882 898 898
+4407342408967

ISBN: 978-93-6452-653-1

Cover design: Shivani
Typesetting: Sagar

First Edition: August 2024

*To the metamorphosis of our journeys...*
*Because she is real and forever...*
*Because she says...*
*'The road to success is always under construction'*

# Contents

*Preface – Author in the Making* ............................................. 1
*About – Let's Walk Though* .................................................... 8
*Segment 1: 'P' - Person* ........................................................... 9
   A - Who we are? ..................................................... 10
   B – The Crossroads ................................................ 13
   C – Relationships and You ..................................... 15
   D – The Bonding Roots .......................................... 18
   E - Mapping Happiness with Expectations ............. 20
   F - Under-confidence ............................................. 23
   G – Oh! Perfect Life ............................................... 26
   H – The Time Wasters ........................................... 28
   I - The Story of Day and Night ............................... 29
   J – The Treasured Soap .......................................... 30
   K - The Story of Value Creation ............................. 32
*Segment II: 'P' – Profession* .................................................. 34
   A – First Impressions ............................................. 35
   B - The Journey of Self Integration ......................... 38
   C - Team Power ..................................................... 41
   D - Top 10 Tools for Impactful Communication ...... 44
   E - Leadership and Collaborative Instincts ............. 46
   F- Buckets of an Impactful Profile .......................... 49
   G - Interview Hygiene Checks ................................ 59
   H- The C-A-R Concept ........................................... 66
   I - Unfolding Stakeholder Harmony ........................ 69
   J - Your Transferable's ........................................... 72

  K - Emma's Mid-Career Era ......................................... 75

*Segment III –A: Student Community Special* ................... 80
  A - Unlocking Academic Excellence ......................... 80
  B - Top Skill Spots for a Lucrative Profession ............. 84
  C - Work and Vocals go hand-in-hand ....................... 89
  D - Seven Step Guide to Choosing your
  MBA Program ......................................................... 93
  E- Setting your base for Finance, Marketing and Human Resource Functions ................................................... 97
  F - Media and Content Mantras ............................. 104

*Segment III – B: Self Care Series* ........................................ 116
  A - Staying in Sync with nature .............................. 117
  B - Art of Mind Cleansing ...................................... 122
  C - Upgrading Your Sub-Conscious ......................... 125
  D - The 4 R Tool ..................................................... 127
  E - Freedom within or without boundaries? ............... 130
  F - Early Bird Realizations ....................................... 133
  G - Reflections, my piece of life... ........................... 135

*About the Author:* ................................................................. 137

# *Preface – Author in the Making*

What and how we feel, stems from every moment of truth we experience during our lives. Some fade away and some stay. But, one from the many becomes a dream turn true. This piece is dedicated to my dream turn reality.

I remember my dad always telling me, "If you have a place for one chapatti, take only one. If you take two, someone will be left with none."

While entering college, I told dad that I wanted to do pedicure, he put me on to a beautician training short course and said, "complete the program and go ahead with your pedicure".

I learnt the difference between 'need' and 'want' well in time. Almost nothing came easy but I was generally a happy soul from a closely bonded nuclear family. Free-hours would find me with storybooks instead of Barbie houses.

Time flew by, but the one constant that remained with me was books. From Comics to Nancy Drews to Agatha Christies to The Roadless Travelled to the Stephen Coveys to the Daile Carnegies' of the world.

Within three days of completing my graduation exam, I landed a job. Never to look back, I walked - I fell - I stood up. Again, I walked - I fell - I stood up....

Around fifteen years ago, a normal fight-patch up gift from a dear friend was this book. Reading being my first love as always, I started with it.

The opening line said, "The road to success is always under construction."

Here is the thing - It was not just a book!

The author was talking to me. Each line was just what I needed. There was tremendous gravity. Somewhere, deep within, I felt belonged. Less than halfway through, I could well understand why the book was titled what it was.

'Come On! GET SET GO' had almost started wrapping my tears and smiles at every step. Sometimes, I would wonder if I would ever be able to meet this author in person and tell her what she and her book meant to me.

While I had never really aspired for more than a stable profession and a secured roof with a handful of honest people around, God had decided to be kind. Just that wish to meet the author lingered within.

Cut to three years ago, around mid – 2021, a lady with the same name as the author joined as the director in one of the major departments of the organization I was working with.

I did come across her during some of the common office meetings, but COVID being in the season, we were masks on; so she just remained as someone with the same name.

On 9th January 2022, day two of my COVID, I was burning with a 104-degree fever and the agony of a thousand needles pierced in my body.

Isolated and crying in pain to myself, at 2.00p.m. my WhatsApp beeped, "How are you feeling, Aditi?" I replied, "Will get better." The next message said, "You are a brave girl."

Who was this person asking about my well-being, like having known me but I do not have the number saved, nor do I know the name?

The message had a very strong and familiar vibe, but who was it? I chose to see the display picture of this well-wisher. It felt familiar, but I was not able to gather who it was.

One Saturday, a few days after my RCPTR report tested negative, I was clearing up my room. I picked up, GET SET GO for another much-needed read.

The realisation struck! The face on the cover page of the book and the WhatsApp display picture looked similar.

I checked to compare. Again, and again. I showed it to my parents and my neighbours to be sure. They said just what I longed to hear.

The next morning, when I saved her number, I realized that she was part of my workplace WhatsApp group. I felt sensitive to the gravity I was experiencing but was extremely unsure.

Is this author the same as her books? Or is she different? Should I tell her? Should I not?

A fortnight later, when I was swiping in at the office, I saw a big blue car come in and stop near the swipe machine. The driver ran out to open the door and a lady stepped out. She had not fixed her mask then.

Graceful as ever, her face reflected peace. Her eyes signified truth. Her forehead personified originality. Each step she took was thoroughly thoughtful.

She smiled at me. I was shivering with nervousness but I greeted her back. We walked towards the lift. I stepped back to let her get in first but she held my hand and took me along.

My eyes were moist with tears though I did manage to hide them from her. She was my GET SET GO!

It took me nearly six months to tell her that I had read her books and what she and GET SET GO meant to me.

Though we belonged to two different worlds, conversations helped us get to know each other bit by bit, with both, – gaps and no gaps put-together.

She was a hard task master but cotton soft from within, no different from her books. She inspired me to listen to my inner being and connected me to my core.

I started scribbling on to blogs, from zero then to 70 plus now. I would ask her insights on the making of her books, how the ideas would come to her, the research and thought- flow adapted.

She would help me polish up my writing and guide me towards the depth of my being with various integrities of life and much more. She unfolded me into an Aditi I never knew.

She extended me, the soft copy of her book, '360-Degree Excel' while it was in the publish phase, even before it had touched the distribution market. I still remember the excitement of reading it overnight and the emotion of being able to express your thoughts about your favourite author's book to the author herself.

She gave me a copy of her poetry book, 'Ek Baat Teri – Ek Baat Meri', which she had co-authored with her husband. It was not on the sale track at that point and was one of her two written pieces I had not read amongst all her other books.

She did share some of its making, as to how she framed the answers first and questions were formed later by the co-author.

The tender flavour of her thoughts and its sync with the actionable was life-affirming!

Humble, reciprocating, understanding, and transparent, she would place me in a comfortable zone to handle whatever came.

I remember when the top floor of my building caught fire last year and we had to vacate it with immediate effect, I was out of home for almost two weeks. She made sure to send me meals daily. Just like a mom, she would ask, "Will you have dal-dhokli tomorrow?"

We shared so much in common, from the karela's and the undhiyu's to the boondi raitas and the patra's to the soups to the khichdi's to the dal dhokli's to the infinities of our thoughts and actions.

The origin being - our bonding through books, to our conversations, to her aura, and her gestures and the feeling of care I was experiencing towards her.

She would hold me settle the tiniest of my discomforts. I felt vulnerable like never before and somewhere a little fear of getting used to her.

My journey from a stranger to being invited to the heights of her home was genuinely beautiful. A sacred experience - treasured for life!

I eventually realized her deep presence in my space and I do understand that I may not be the only Aditi in her world.

This middle-class normal being called 'Aditi,' who is from your local neighbourhood in Mumbai, did meet her favourite author to live what had felt belonged.

The thought, the connecting dots and the courage to align 'Let's Walk- Through' in to a book comes to me from My GET SET GO, Dr. Swati Lodha.

Dr. Swati Lodha is a #1 bestselling author, educationist, leadership, and parenting expert, think tank for senior citizens' wisdom and ageism, serial social entrepreneur, coach, motivational speaker, and a mom. She has bagged dozens of awards in her career, spanning of over 24 years and has transformed lives, coached more than 10k plus corporate executives and young minds.

Her LinkedIn Profile: **linkedin.com/in/drswatilodha**

Most importantly, she is a simple human with an honest heart. I am truly grateful to her for nurturing and giving birth to an author in me.

# About – Let's Walk Though

'Let's Walk Through' is a pen down of raw thoughts, stories, and experiential elements with a hope that it partners you while you navigate your walk through from your heart and mind to paper, person and profession.

It has been written as a gentle reminder of how our core habits, mindset, behaviour, and attitude towards the situation's life presents us with, effect the directions of our journey and can change almost everything.

It seeks to hand hold us with things that are minor yet essential for one's inner growth and sense of contentment as a person and in the professional space.

Let's Walk Through aims to share insights on how we tend to ignore them just because we hold on to our own notions more dearly.

This book aims to serve as partner towards a progressive life envisaged by us for ourself with an effort of a little more than 100%.

Going forward, I request you to read each capsule, sync in, relate it to an instance that matters or mattered to you and shape it up to the direction you envisage.

Ultimately, 'Learn – Unlearn – Relearn' is what our journeys define themselves as...

# Segment 1: 'P' - Person

# A - Who we are?

There was a king who mindfully ruled a huge happy empire. He always demonstrated value for progressive people and occurrences. One day a portrait carver came to his palace with three beautiful full-length human portraits for sale. The portraits were mesmerizing, created of marble, with great detailing. Eyes, nose, facial features, expressions, and body structure; so amazing that it made them look real.

The king melted looking at them and decided to purchase one. So, he asked the carver, "What is the cost?" The carver said, "The 1st one cost Rs. 5000, the 2nd one is worth fifty thousand and the third one is two lakh fifty thousand rupees". The king was stunned by the massive price difference as all three portraits looked the same.

He asks his team of ministers to find out why the vast difference in cost. What was it with the portrait that cost 2.5 lakh?

One by one, all the cabinet members checked, touched, felt, and smelled each of the portraits trying to identify the difference that had affected the cost so much. None of them could identify the difference.

Finally, the kind called his most intelligent minister and told him to find out the reason for the cost difference.

This minister had a look at all the three portraits carefully and asked his subordinate to get three small pearls.

He put one pearl in one ear of the first portrait. After a few moments that pearl dropped out from the 2nd ear.

Then he went to the second portrait and put a pearl in his ear. This pearl dropped out of the portrait's mouth in around half an hour.

He then went to the third portrait and put a pearl in his ear. He waited. This time the pearl did not come out. It had synced in.

The minister then told the king, " Sir, I found the difference."

Everyone in the assembly including the king was extremely curious to know the finding!

The minister said, "The first portrait listened and took in everything that came from one ear but threw it out from the other. The second one also took in what came but narrated it to everyone around. He did not absorb and self-imply. Hence both dropped the pearl out. The 3rd portrait took in what came, absorbed the learning experiences from it and did not drop it out like the first two. That was the unique quality which placed him high at value as compared to the others."

In one of her books, Dr. Swati Lodha talks about the three kinds of women but I chose to call it humans, one who lives inside the well, one who stays in a web and one with a well inside.

The 1st one lives in a submissive format, the 2nd is confused forever and the third type is a thoughtful human who comes alive to every moment.

My piece of thought here is who we are and what do we desire to be?

# B – The Crossroads

Human life is like a train travel journey. Every age and crossroad of life is a station, where the journey takes a momentary halt. There are these arrivals and departures of people and situations at the halts. It is god's way of telling you that the roles are over or then there is yet a station more to travel.

Everything is with and for a purpose, known - unknown. That purpose passes through a phase of independence, and walks out at the next halt.

If not, the purpose then travels through the journey of dependence. This is the riskiest phase as expectations develop, just like spilt ends in healthy hair. A lot of departures happen here.

And those that do not; reach the road to inter-dependence., the safest and the healthiest.

A 50 -50 equation with both people and situations. Not all but you do have a small percentage of control in your hand, as to the shape you want the journey to take. But that is only possible when you are in control of yourself.

You also in many instances need to decide what matters to you more...

Situations? Topics? Or People? Or then your peace of mind? Hold on to what matters.

It is not always necessary to have a last word even if you know you have a valid perspective. That does not mean that you do not speak up for something that affects you.

Sometimes it consumes an entire life to understand a simple ABC. Do not be surprised if that experience comes to you. Just remember to be responsible for your thoughts and actions.

And the rest will follow...

## C – Relationships and You...

As human beings, as social beings, there is this one thing that is a default element of our life.

Yes - Relationships. With Yourself, Your family, Your friends and peers, Your classmates and colleagues, Your mentors and bosses, Your besties, and Your life partners. They are not all.

You also do have a relationship with your surroundings, nature, pets, food, daily use-ables and lots more.

In short, your relationships are with both, human and non-human elements. Defined and Undefined. With and Without Labels.

Complex right? I feel it is like a pizza - always confusing, it comes in a square box, and when you open it, it is round. And when you go to eat it, the pieces are triangular.

Life and People are also like a pizza - look different, appear different and behave completely different!

Remember, we as humans live one of the strongest relationships that is the one you have with yourself. That is the relationship that last you the longest and remains at its peak lifelong.

But does it mean that we do not need or should not maintain any other human relationships.

We must. We should. We need! After all, we are social beings. We do love-hate, smile - sob, share - care and all of it. And that is in majority because of our relationship with others.

Across the human relationships that we share, we understand who matters to us and who does not. Of course, there is a chance of you being important to someone but that did not show up in recent occurrences.

Besides, every person has a different way of expressing and our ability to understand the expressions vary.

There may or may not be a match in both. However, such situations do affect us, irrespective of how strong or mature we appear to be or are.

It is very important to be mindful of the time and thought you invest in someone. A relationship cannot and should not be measured through ROI alone but it should be worth your investment.

Every time that someone matters to you or you matter to someone, does not mean you need to keep reminding or keep being reminded that you are important or will be reciprocated all the while.

But keeping the communication alive helps one to know how the other person is feeling. Most of the times this is exactly what goes unnoticed.

Yes, those expressions are crucial but hold value only when expressed at the right time, with right people and in the right situation.

By being worth your investment, it means you have learnt something from the relationship. It has made you stronger, tolerant, less judgemental, and lesser cry-baby or developed you in some way.

For me, I became emotionally rich. Yes, that relationship has given me tears and made me experience difficult emotions. But the truth is, without that discomfort, it is impossible to have these value ads happen to me.

Value Ads, not in material but as an individual. True Relationships are HARD, that is probably why they are extremely beautiful.

# D –The Bonding Roots

In a small township amidst rolling hills, there lived a young boy named Samir. He was unlike any other child in his neighbourhood; his heart overflowed with boundless love for his parents, Sameera and Sawaan. On a crisp autumn day, as the golden leaves danced in the breeze, his school held its 'Annual Career Day Event.'

Each student was asked, "What do you want to become when you grow up?"

While his classmates dreamt of becoming astronauts, doctors, or fire-fighters, Samir had a different aspiration.

He penned his response on the exam paper, "I want to become a mobile so that I can stay in my father's hands. So that my mother can look at me and smile. I want to become an instrument that will stay in their hands all the time, so they will be happy spending time with me".

Little did anyone know; these words carried the weight of Samir's deepest desires.

As Sameera and Sawaan, a hardworking labourer couple read their son's answer; tears welled up in their eyes. They realized the depth of their son's love and the sacrifices he was willing to make to bring them joy.

Moved beyond words, Sameera and Sawaan embraced him tightly, showering him with love and gratitude. From that moment on, they cherished every moment spent with him, realizing that his presence was the greatest gift of all.

Years passed, and Samir grew into a compassionate and caring young man.

Though life presented its challenges, the bond between Samir and his parents remained unbreakable. Through every triumph and turbulence they stood together, their love unwavering and pure.

And so, in the quiet corners of that little town, the story of Samir's heartfelt answer echoed through the years, reminding all who heard it of the power of love and the beauty of selflessness.

For in the end, it is not the grandeur of our aspirations that defines us, but the depth of our love and the connections we hold close to our hearts.

# E - Mapping Happiness with Expectations

I was speaking to an old friend the other day. She was discussing some crucial personal elements. While journaling later that night, I reflected on our conversation, how and what happiness has to do with expectations.

I asked myself - what is happiness? It is purely a state of mind, what we are thinking or feeling at a particular moment.

I may have everything and still not be happy or then have nothing and still be fine. Alot of us, without realizing it, stay in a permanent chase mode, in an ongoing want spree.

This project - That dress - This resort- That Car- This Award - Those targets.

We always want, thinking it will give us happiness. But the truth is that most of the time, deep within we are not sure if getting that want is going to make us happy.

Pro-Tip: The 'why' of our want needs to be in place to set the rest right. Chances are whatever we are chasing; our goals or expectations are not ours at all.

We should first figure out the strings of our expectations.

- Expectations others have from us. Our relationships - Parents, Siblings, Spouses, Friends and more.
- Our expectations from others. We want a friend or our parents to understand us.
- There is a third type and trust me – it is a genuine disaster!

It is our expectations of ourselves because we think others have those expectations from us. A child believes that his parents want him to stand first in class.

So, he must achieve that to make his parents proud. That becomes his chase mode. When such an expectation of ourselves remains unfulfilled, it leads to unhappiness.

My teenager who likes to stay in simple attire, when she sees family members dress up well, she starts thinking that dressing up well is what is expected from her. So, there is this constant burden to be someone else, to be the version she is supposed to be.

Similarly, if I am happy at home and my best friend who is a travel freak says, "You will realize only when you move out."

This happens to seem like an expectation from my friend on what or who I should be.

Pro-Tip: Understand that the 'Should be you' is not or may not be the you, that you want to become.

That is the 'you' others want you to be or then you envisage that others want you to be. The best deal would be to be what your core.

Anything beyond would be like trying to make compartments of water!

To figure out our core, first, we need to get there. For instance - who is Aditi? What defines her as a person?

Well, 'People and situations will come and go, but you will need you.'

The key is to Accept. Accept Your Core and let the existing fluidity remain.

Go with the flow while we alter the path in a need-based format. This is something only we can do for our self.

## F- Under-Confidence

We come across several situations during our lives - home - study -work. Not all of them will be happy and that is given!

The one common element across is Under-confidence. Most of the time we end up feeling insecure because of others, while they are not sure themselves.

I still remember an instance from my graduation years. One day one, a professor asked our class, "Who of you doesn't feel confident?".

While there was pin drop silence, one student from the last bench stood up to say, "Ma'am, I don't feel safe to share my opinions here. I feel scared of being judged".

I can never forget how our class gave her a huge round of applause for that statement. The entire class could relate to what she said!

In my experience, three factors mainly contribute to Under-confidence

The first 'D' of Under-confidence is Doubt.

That is when you do not believe in yourself. I have seen so many people with already decided stuff about themselves. "I am not good enough. She looks so much better. I do not talk as fluently as her".

I am sure, all of us can resonate. This results from a lack of being able to validate your core, self-validation and our need for being the popular, external-validation.

When it does not reach us right is because we see our actions from "OPP"- Other People's Perspective.

We must remember that we cannot make everyone happy all the time! And it is completely okay.

Pro-tip: Everyone is not meant to know everything or be happy all the time.

The next 'D' of Under-confidence is Discourage. We humans are our own biggest enemies. I know it does not sound proper but unfortunately, it is the hard truth!

We are rarely kind to ourselves and tend to feel that we may never be able to do a thing we desire in future because we are unable to do it now.

Pro-tip: Each ill need not have a pill. There is no need to be discouraged!

You may not be apt at something today but can learn with consistent efforts and some patience. I find it funny today but a couple of years ago, we cousins decided to meet for a week-long fun trip. It was my first time travelling by air and I was super nervous. I kept telling people around, "It's my first trip by air, oh first time."

The anxiety was so high that I went and stood in the wrong queue. The floor attendant guided me to the correct cue. I told almost everyone about what was happening and kept repeating.

One of my cousins took me to the side and said, "Aditi, relax. Do not get so anxious. You have over-told your story. Even the people who did not know, now know that you stood in the wrong queue."

That was the 3rd 'D' of Under-confidence – Diminish.

I say this with confidence as someone who has been there and knows how it feels.

Pro-tip: Never Diminish yourself. A first time will always be there and it can be weird.

# G – Oh! Perfect Life

A dear friend when asked about her well-being said "Oh I have a perfect life.", Well. honestly, I am happy for her. But the truth is that the definition of perfection is very subjective.

It is like saying, "This dress material is of good quality". Here good quality refers to nothing but fit to use. The fit-to-use elements are different for different people. Besides, nothing is ever perfect, neither life nor mankind.

The day we wake up thinking that the entire day is going to be seamless, trust me there will be a trace of glitch somewhere.

When we as humans are conscious of our expectations, imbalances are negligible. When an imbalance is negligible, we are in control of ourselves and content with what life gives us. That is because our 'Needs' are aligned and in sync.

When we accept this, we can build up to our 'Wants' based on our capacity. And just in case we are unable to reach our 'Wants', the imbalance does not trouble us because we well-understand the difference between a 'Need' and 'Want'.

"Oh, I have a perfect life with absolutely no drama. It just cannot be more perfect" - Well. Even this sounds dramatic!

Because it is difficult to figure whether we are trying to convince ourselves or the person we are telling this to.

Drama is an integral and unavoidable part of human life. Every life has drama; else it would not be life at all - birth, death, breathing, sunrise, sunset smile, tears, season, pain, joy, and sorrow.

All of this that every human perceives as a natural course of life. Imagine, if drama would not exist, there would be no difference between a table - chair and a human being.

Once we are in alignment with our needs and wants, we learn to just stay normal and make no efforts to show any perfectness or then sound over-happy.

What it is, will just be natural and normal. The catch arises only if negativity creeps in. It is important to be alert and maintain distance from negativity of every form. That is when we need to say 'No'.

So, No Drama Please! Or, Oh! Drama Please?

# H – The Time Wasters

Mr. Donkey and Mr. Tiger were debating on the grass being green. Mr. Donkey insisted that the grass was blue while Mr. Tiger kept saying it was green. After a lot of arguments about it, both went to Mr. Lion, the king of the forest. Mr. Tiger complained to Mr. Lion that Mr. Donkey was arguing with him that the grass was blue, when it is not. Mr. Donkey got hyper about it and told Mr. Lion that he should be punished because the grass is blue, not green!

Mr. Lion announced a punishment for Mr. Tiger, 'Silence for 12 months'. Mr. Donkey was overjoyed and continued back on his way, singing and dancing. Mr. Tiger, disappointed and unhappy with this asked Mr. Lion about the punishment despite the truth being grass is green.

Mr. Lion said to Mr. Tiger, "Punishment has nothing to do with the grass being blue or green. In fact, it is green."

In response, Mr. Tiger asked Mr. Lion, "Then why the punishment to me?" Mr. Lion replied, "Because you wasted your time arguing and trying to convince Mr. Donkey and to top that you wasted my time, expecting me to address the issue when the universe knows that the grass is green, and it doesn't matter whether Mr. Donkey agrees to it or not."

# 1 - The Story of Day and Night

A lady gave birth to twin girls. One of them was white as snow and the other was dark as night. Neighbours, friends, and acquaintances would show their preference towards the fair girl and ignore the other. They would also make fun of her owing to her dark complexion.

Eventually, the fair girl was called 'Day' and the dark one was labelled as 'Night'.

'Night' would feel very hurt when she was ignored and laughed at due to her skin colour.

She would cry when alone many a times. Deeply pained, one day she decided to go away somewhere and left her home.

Her family and friends initially thought she would come back. But for more than a month she did not. Now there was only 'Day', 24*7 without the 'Night'.

So, people had to only work and work without time for peace, rest, or sleep without the calm and soothing effect of the moon.

People started realising that only 'Day' without 'Night' were not what it was meant to be.

They wanted 'Night' to come back. Both 'Day' and 'Night' were needed to complete the cycle of each date, month, and year.

Without a smile, we do not realise the worth of a tear. And without a tear, we do not value a smile. And without both together, life does not align in sync....

# J – The Treasured Soap

Have you ever felt like giving up? That breaking point is when you feel like you have tried everything and yet, nothing seems to work.

Whether it is at work, in studies, or in a relationship, we've all been there. Many of us are, even now!

But wait...read on, carefully before you choose to lose hope...

There was a girl who was a die-hard government job aspirant. She did not care about the role or department - all she wanted was to be a government employee.

She made her first attempt of the exam for government job and failed.

Second attempt - failed.

Third attempt - failed.

Fourth attempt - failed.

Year after year, she kept preparing and giving exams until she reached the last year where she could attempt the exam in terms of eligibility.Can you imagine the pressure she must have felt to be on that last chance point?

But she did not give up. She took all her struggles, failures, and bounce backs, and decided to attempt the exam one last time.

And this time... she cleared it, finally getting a government job in a good organization.

She clicked a picture of all the scribbled books and papers she had used for all those years of struggle. The ink of the multiple dozens of pens got over but her spirit stayed alive.

I have seen the journeys of many people, success, failure, and rejection, but never have I seen a person's entire journey of effort, downfall, and bounce backs all captured in one single click.

The moral of the story is that you may fail a million times, but never let the failure define you.

If you do not fail, you will never learn, and if you do not learn, you will never experience success.

A hard truth - success stems out of failure. A harder truth, the definition of success needs to essentially be your own.

## K- The Story of Value Creation

A good friend of mine would misplace his writing pens very often. He would buy only cheap ones so it would not bother him if he lost a pen and needed to buy a new one. The only thing he was worried about was his habit.

The Habit of being careless as he felt.

One day, I suggested him to buy the most expensive pen possible and see what would happen. He did that and purchased a 22-carat gold pen.

After nearly six months, I spoke to him last week

I asked him if he continued to lose the pens?

The answer was - No.

He told me that he is very careful with his costly pen.

He said, himself is surprised as to how the change happened.

I told him that the value of the pen made the difference and there was nothing wrong with him in person.

This is what happens in our life also. We are careful with the things that we value the most.

If we value our life and health, we will be careful about what and how we eat, and look after ourselves by adequately nurturing our mind, body, and soul.

If we value our near and dear ones, we will treasure our relationships.

If we value resources and money we will utilise it mindfully.

If we value our time, we will use it constructively rather than waste it.

If we value living beings, we will be extra careful and treat them with respect.

If we value nature, we will make sure we do not exploit it.

Most of the time's we realise the value of people, resources, and situations only after losing them or when we understand the threat that we are on the verge of losing them.

# Segment II: 'P' – Profession

# A – First Impressions

In the bustling city of Mumbai, nestled among towering skyscrapers, lay the headquarters of a well-known MNC. Pallavi Goir, freshly completed her masters, nervously adjusted her blazer as she stepped into the sleek lobby.

She was about to embark on her first day as a management trainee. The receptionist greeted her warmly, directing her to the elevator that would whisk her to the 20th floor.

As the doors opened, she entered a hive of activity. People rushed past, heads buried in laptops or engaged in intense discussions.

Pallavi took a deep breath, steeling herself for the challenges ahead. Her manager, Mr. Gopal Narang, welcomed her with a firm handshake and a kind smile.

He introduced her to the team—a mix of seasoned professionals and bright-eyed post-graduates like herself.

They exchanged pleasantries, but Pallavi could sense their curiosity and scrutiny. The first task assigned to Pallavi was to study the brand and present her innovative ideas to optimize its promotion and visibility to the next level.

Feeling the weight of responsibility, she immersed herself in the study.

Hours passed like minutes as she delved deep into the intricacies of the brand life cycle. As the sun dipped below the skyline, Pallavi found the elusive but - like an untouched stone buried deep within the brand USP.

With her heart pounding, she patched the code and designed her deck. She researched heavily on the role of its implementation. Her presentation was a super success!

News of Pallavi's accomplishment spread like wildfire through the office. Her colleagues praised her diligence and insights. Mr. Gopal commended her during the team meeting, highlighting her contribution to the project's success.

Pallavi blushed with pride, realizing she had made a positive impression right on her first day. In the weeks that followed, Pallavi continued to excel. She collaborated seamlessly with her team, eagerly absorbing knowledge from her more experienced colleagues, and aligned her KRA's beautifully.

Her confidence grew, and soon she was leading her own projects, making significant contributions to the company's growth. Reflecting on her journey, Pallavi understood the importance of first impressions.

By demonstrating her skills, work ethic, and eagerness to learn, she had earned the respect and trust of her peers.

Each day was a new challenge, but Pallavi faced them head-on, knowing she had established herself as a valuable member of the team from day one.

Often, a dignified and graceful dressing can leave a lasting first impression. It communicates that you value yourself and your role, which can positively influence how others perceive your competence and reliability.

Dressing and communicating with proactive clarity and confidence play crucial roles in creating a positive impact at the office, influencing how one is perceived and respected by colleagues and superiors alike.

Ultimately, the communication of your clothes holds equal importance in the impact value as your own.

Both put together contribute to establishing credibility, fostering relationships, and enhancing overall productivity and success in the workplace.

## B- The Journey of Self Integration

When I was drafting this piece, I realised that I was getting distracted mid-way and was not able to concentrate at all.

A flood of varying thoughts showering at the same time and some of the capsules of this segment refuse to get a closure for weeks together! In this hustle - bustle, I found myself overwhelmed, juggling multiple thoughts and tasks, I realized something had to change. That something was managing myself for optimized productivity.

I am sure you also some point would surely have had a situation where you felt that you are trying hard to do something but are not able to.

Here is what I did, and it helps...

The first step, I took was to define clear, crisp actionable goals. I started by identifying what I wanted to achieve. This clarity helped me prioritize and allocate my time effectively.

For instance, instead of saying "I want to increase sales", set a specific goal like, "I will increase sales by 20% in the next quarter by implementing a new marketing strategy."

With a myriad of tasks competing for my attention, I adopted prioritization techniques and it helped me distinguish between urgent and important tasks, allowing me to focus on what truly mattered.

What I also mean here is to identify your distracters and minimize them. This could mean turning off notifications, finding a quiet workspace, or using productivity apps to block distracting websites. Implementing time blocking mechanism proved a game-changer for me. By dedicating specific blocks of time to different tasks or projects, I minimized distractions and maintained momentum throughout the day.

Stay present in the moment and focus on one task at a time. Mindfulness Techniques such as deep breathing or meditation can help calm your mind, improve concentration, re-energize your brain, and enhance focus.

Break your work into intervals, time set for focused work followed by a short break. This technique helps maintain productivity while preventing burnout.

Set a timer for 25 minutes and work on a specific task without any distractions. After the timer goes off, take a 5-minute break to stretch, grab a snack, or simply rest your eyes.

Leveraging technology tools like task management apps and calendar integrations helped me stay organized and informed. Automating routine tasks freed up mental space for more productive outcomes.

Self-management is not a one-time achievement but a continuous process of learning and adaptation.

I regularly reflect on my progress, adjust strategies as needed, and remain open to new productivity methods.

Most importantly, I learnt that self-management extends far beyond productivity. It also involves prioritizing self-care, setting boundaries, and nurturing relationships.

Incorporating mindfulness practices and regular exercise into my routine boosted my resilience and overall happiness.

Finally, accountability and support were crucial in maintaining momentum. I sought mentorship and surrounded myself with a supportive network that encouraged my growth and held me accountable for my goals.

Moral of the story: Through intentional efforts and perseverance, I can align balance in my life by adapting a multidimensional approach. Start small, stay committed, and celebrate every milestone along the way.

Pro -Tip: "You can't control the monsoons of life, but you can surely create an umbrella raincoat for yourself!"

# C-Team Power

Last month my graduation college invited me for an alumni interaction. The focus was to convince the students to volunteer with an NGO catering to orphan children as they were the batch of would - be-sociology graduates.

This initiative also needed them to gather donation to the tune of rupees 10/- per head by approaching various educational institutions and communicating to students there.

As I stepped into the packed classroom buzzing with restless energy, I could sense a mix of curiosity and distraction among the students.

Some were eager to leave, others fidgeted in discomfort, a few looked hungry, and many looked bored with the thought of another speech!

Amidst this sea of faces, one girl caught my eye. She looked at me, giggled, and whispered to her friend.

I straightened my clothes and hair nervously before beginning, just to tone down my self-consciousness.

"Hello everyone," I started, trying to sound confident. "I am here to talk about something important." Their attention wavered, so I decided to try something different.

"Let's try an experiment," I suggested, with a hint of excitement. I asked one of the last benchers, "What is your name please"?

She said, "Divyanka". I requested her to come out, stand next to me, and shout her name aloud.

Divyanka, a bit unsure, came out, next to me and exclaimed her name. I asked her to repeat it, louder this time. The class watched, amused.

"Now, everyone," I announced, "On the count of three, shout your names together!"

A chorus of names filled the room, echoing off the walls. The effect was immediate—the students looked surprised at the collective sound they had created.

"Just like that," I continued, seizing the moment. "Your voices together are powerful. Just as one voice stood out, imagine what happens when we combine our efforts."

Initially, the idea of donating just 10 rupees each seemed trivial. But the vocal action painted a picture. "Imagine, if everyone here contributed. It's not just about the money—it's about showing that together, we can create something meaningful."

The room fell silent as they pondered on the action and what I tried telling them. The message was sinking in.

"Each one of you matters," I said, "and together, we can make a real difference for those in need. It's not about the amount but it is about the unity and impact we create when we work together."

I could see thoughtful expressions and exchanged glances among the students. They were beginning to see the power of collective action.

I continued, "Your communication to students of the institutions you visit could be on similar lines or you can create your premise that serves the purpose."

Remember – Team Power matters.

# D- Top 10 Tools for Impactful Communication

In the previous capsule, I shared a story of my alumni interaction session at my graduation college, emphasizing on team power. Taking the same forward, let us delve into the Top Ten Tools for High-Impact Communication:

- Confidence and Clarity: Ensure you are confident and clear about your topic; this naturally enhances the power of your speech.
- Use of Facts and Engagement: Incorporate facts, figures, and interactive elements like calling out names or involving listeners in activities like I requested Divyanka for her name exclaim. This keeps your talk authentic and your audience engaged.
- Effective Gestures: can significantly enhance communication. Remember the girl who caught my eye with a subtle gesture during my talk?
- Speak with Conviction: Start with a strong statement or an exciting experiment setting the tone for your discussion. This strengthens your message.
- Storytelling: Use storytelling techniques to paint vivid pictures in your listeners' minds.

Even without graphics, words like "10 rupee note" or inviting someone like Divyanka to participate can create powerful mental images.

- Engage Audience's Imagination: Encourage your audience to visualize your narrative through gestures and compelling storytelling with actionable, names, places, situations, objects...
- Stimulate Thought: Engage your audience with activities or discussions relevant to the environment, as I did by sensing the restlessness in the class.
- Foster Personalization: Customize your talk using inclusive language (e.g., "we," "I", "you") instead of distancing terms like "they."
- Use of Relatable Examples: Use personal anecdotes to make your message more relatable, may be like what I did experiences from alumni interactions depending on the reference to the context of your talk.
- Actionable Insights: Demonstrate concepts through examples or actionable insights, illustrating how individual and collective voices can create impact.

Communication aims to inform, entertain, or act out - choose your approach based on your intended purpose.

# E- Leadership and Collaborative Instincts

In the heart of a 24 by 7 life-full city, there was a small community centre called 'Harmony Home'. It was a place where people from diverse backgrounds came together to learn, grow, and support each other.

Milli, a passionate and empathetic leader at Harmony Home, was known for her unwavering belief in the power of collaboration. She believed that true leadership was not about authority but about fostering an environment where everyone's strengths could shine.

One chilly autumn afternoon, a storm brewed over the city, bringing torrential rain and gusty winds that rattled windows and sent leaves swirling through the streets.

Inside Harmony Home, a crisis was unfolding. The roof, weakened by years of wear, began to leak profusely, threatening to damage the premises.

Milli gathered her team—a group of volunteers and staff members with diverse skills and backgrounds—and presented the challenge.

"We need to fix the roof quickly to protect our home," she announced, her voice firm yet filled with determination.

Among the team was Mainak, a retired engineer with a knack for problem-solving, and Sarah, a young artist known for her creativity and resourcefulness.

Together with others, they brainstormed ideas, pooled their resources, and divided tasks efficiently. Mainak assessed the damage while Sarah gathered materials donated by local businesses.

As they worked tirelessly through the night, a spirit of camaraderie and purpose infused their efforts.

Each person brought something unique to the table—whether it was technical expertise, artistic flair, or organizational skills.

They communicated openly, listened actively, and respected each other's ideas, guided by steady encouragement and belief in their abilities.

Outside, the storm raged on, but inside Harmony Home, a different kind of storm was weathered—a storm of challenges turned into opportunities, of individual efforts woven into a tapestry of collective achievement.

Days turned into weeks as the repairs progressed. News of their endeavour spread through the community, drawing support from neighbours and local businesses alike.

People volunteered their time, skills, and resources, inspired by the unity and purpose displayed at Harmony Home.

Finally, the day arrived when the last nail was hammered in place, and the roof stood strong and secure once more.

The team gathered beneath it, weary but triumphant, their faces glowing with pride. Milli stood among them, her eyes shining with gratitude. "This wasn't just about fixing a roof," she said, her voice echoing through the now-silent room.

"It was about coming together as a community, leveraging our strengths, and showing what can be achieved when we work together."

The story of Harmony Home and its resilient community spread far and wide, becoming a testament to the transformative power of leadership, and collaborative skills.

Milli's belief that leadership is not about standing above others but standing with them has not only saved a building but also strengthened the bonds of a community, proving that when people unite with a shared vision, they can overcome any storm that comes their way.

# F- Buckets of an Impactful Profile

The most crucial part of your career journey is the start point, Your Profile. We may feel it is just one or two sheets of paper.

But no! Here is the thing:

The journey of your resume starts very early in life. Over and above the routine academic and cultural activities during undergraduate college tenure, teenagers must be encouraged to use the vacation time constructively by doing short internships, taking additional training in utility functions like writing, public speaking, office automation, and presentation tools like advanced excel, power point and keynote amongst others.

This is an add-on to the resume in terms of experience, knowledge, and certificate value and a support system to a fresher's resume which would otherwise consist of nothing other than personal and educational details or probably a standard four-banana race prize.

Using the undergraduate-level vacation constructively also brings along a lot of maturity, accountability, and clarity of thought in a teenager as to what he or she wants to pursue after graduation.

Which stream to adapt to, whether to move to post-graduation directly or work for a year and then take up higher studies, and so on. Whatever the decision is, it must take into consideration the top five skills the candidate possesses.

Now, how do we do that? The best way is to create a brag sheet.

A brag sheet talks about your achievements and skills with supporting factual examples which you not only speak about during your interview but also add to your resume.

Most important is that those skills and achievements prove of great help in selecting your area of function.

For entry-level candidates, your friends, teachers, and well-wishers could help remind you of various instances and situations where you proved your skills and scored a brownie.

For experienced candidates, a professional network (current or ex-colleagues whom you share a healthy equation with) will be of the best help in building up your brag sheet.

Getting your SWOC analysis crafted with professional support also helps big time!

It is very necessary to understand that an arranged marriage with your profession will always have a higher chance of success and reduce the tendency of divorce.

When you are in the process of selecting your work area, consider your professionally relevant skill sets and the ground realities of the business scenarios of the chosen industry.

Most entry level candidates tend to look at what they are interested in, frame a work area for themselves in their minds and then land up in a situation where they are unable to cope.

That is when the interest levels or the so-called passion seem to fade away like a 1st teenage crush!

The reason being that 'The Real is Different.' This often leaves a bad patch on the candidature and the mind of the individual as well.

Moving to the Resume... It is one of the most important marketing tools of the 'Brand You' when it comes to recruitment.

There are several formats available online and recommended by experts as well. Choose what suits you best but consider ATS compatibility. We will understand more about ATS going forward.

Let us discuss the crucial buckets to create an impactful profile.

A robust profile is not solely defined by academic accolades but also by a well-rounded set of attributes that distinguish one as exceptional.

Craft a concise yet compelling profile summary including your academics, and professional aspirations. If you are uncertain about the domain, maintain a broader outlook initially.

For experienced individuals, this will be an amalgamation of past, current, and futuristic mapped with key skill sets.

A compelling one to hold the interest of the hiring manager. The next subhead will be the Key Highlights which include the major achievements or game changing moments of your journey. Awards, promotions, and performance metric should be added in.

A fresher can add academic or internship related highlights. Next in line are your skills, these are divided into three segments. For example,

- Hard Skills: Marketing, Finance, Content Creation, (domain related).
- Soft Skills: Communication, Networking, Presentation, Collaborative team skills, and the like.
- Technical Know-how: Canva, Advanced Excel, Slides, AI, Chat GPT, Google Forms, SPSS, and other relevant tools.

If your experience is beyond two business cycles, you can term it as 'Key Competencies'.

Back your skills with certifications, projects, job simulations, and internships if you are an entry level candidate.

Remember, if your profile is for your upcoming MBA journey, soft skills come first in the evaluation, next is the hygiene check, I mean the hard skills and the third is your potential.

By potential, here I mean, given your present state, how best you will adapt to the B school learning environment to shape yourself to corporate readiness.

Next in line are your academics, a chronological overview of academics, starting with recent most. Include supplementary diploma courses undertaken to enrich your academic repertoire.

There are ample no cost certifications available on platforms like Management Study Guide, Coursera, Google, HubSpot, Amity Open Learn, LinkedIn and more.

Whether you are a fresher or an experienced professional, relevant up skills are non - negotiable. If you are working or on a sabbatical and can manage the funding, do consider a mid-career change in your academic graph.

For entry level candidates' case studies and competitions prove to be a big time supportive of your skills. Check Olympiads, Unstop and similar portals. This helps hone problem-solving acumen and foster a competitive edge.

For job simulations check Forage, for internships leverage LinkedIn, and do pick up 2 -3 best academic projects. Platforms like Forage not only help in packaging your resume but also aid work domain decision making even before you apply for your first internship.

For MBA evaluation an internship between your TY final exams and the MBA commencement is considered by majority B-Schools for selections.

Positions of Responsibility for entrants highlight notable team and leadership role pursued during college events or committee memberships. Engage in NGO projects, to demonstrate versatility and commitment.

Conclude with pertinent personal information encompassing contact details, date of birth, linguistics, and your updated LinkedIn profile link.

Now that we have got the resume buckets in place, here is to consider a few important tips while you craft your profile.

The client is the king: At this junction, the organisation with an opportunity is your client. Customise the contents of your resume based on the role and the organisation you are applying for.

Fresher's often have very little to customise on, here is when the internships, brag sheets, and additional training are taken come into the picture.

In summary, your resume needs to maintain the curiosity of the recruitment team till they pick up the phone to call you.

Keywords are the Keys....

Most organizations follow the Applicant Tracking Systems (ATS), a tool used to screen relevant profile for the hiring manager to carry out the next steps.

ATS is used majorly when there is a huge count of resumes for a role or then recruitment for multiple roles at a junction. ATS works on mapping keywords in the resume with keywords in the opportunity description to identify apt profiles.

There are ample ATS formats available online or you can check your resume ATS score on online tools like jobs can or resume reworded. It will also suggest the needful changes along with giving you the score.

Keywords are nothing but specific words that match the opportunity requirement and align with the skill set you possess. The use of these makes it easier for the recruiter to shortlist a resume for a particular role.

Being precise: Your resume should be able to tell your work story depending on the nature of the job you have applied for and you're candidature (whether you are applying for an entry-level position or a high-profile role).

For instance, if you mention 'presentation skills' as one of your attributes, let the content of your resume demonstrate the mentioned skill at least once. If you have a year or more of experience you can add up the competencies you have developed spanning the experience.

Be Creative, Consistent, and Resourceful and De-Clutter: The use of standard resume heading sections without info graphic also supports ATS. At the same time, using Header and Footer and Tabular formats does not. It is important to have a font type, size, and paragraph spacing that is legible, consistent, and distinct. Control on Bolds and Italics to ensure maximum impact.

Software's like MS Word have a lot of tools which help in formatting content properly.

Start with latest, be it experience, education, or any other elements of your resume. It means adapting a reverse chronological resume format.

Present what you can bring to the table: Needless to say, a good portfolio is equally important as a crisp resume.

Always try to quantify your achievements as much as possible. It makes your profile feel authentic.

"What can the candidate bring to the table?" is any and every recruiter's first plug point with the increasing dynamics of any business today.

This calls for an impactful demonstration of skill sets by presenting what you have created or strategized.

For example, a scriptwriter's portfolio will need to have at least a dozen short-format and long-format scripts across content genres.

A well-rounded portfolio is of prime importance for every entry-level position. It should ideally contain the best and most relevant academic projects done across graduation and post-graduation as applicable.

Moreover, it should also have a self-learning element, meaning your own creations over and above academics or routines. They could be films, pitch presentations, creative strategies for a brand, re-launch campaigns, trans-media news bulletins or anything else that applies to the work area you are looking at.

For experienced candidates, they would have their past work credentials as well.

Also, note that adding hobbies does not help unless the job role needs it. If I am applying for a marketing role and I add a hobby of watching movies has no relevance unless I apply for a movie marketing role or looking at a production house role.

Hobbies should be planned and put down; sometimes they could be cultivated one's basis of the work you wish to pursue.

But never say, I like reading if you do not mean it!

Use simple, error-free language and avoid jargon, prolonged statements or words that are redundant.

Yes, repetitions are not an effective way of stressing your point, especially for experienced candidates who have had similar job functions across stints. So, avoid repeats. Instead, use keywords.

To summarise, Be the hero of your own story:

Your resume needs to speak about your functional candidature, skills with portfolios to demonstrate them, achievements, qualifications, and experience as applicable.

A one-pager is most effective for up to five years of experience. A maximum of a two-page resume is good to go if you have that kind of content to plug in.

It is a good idea to remember that the human attention span is diminishing by the day!

So, the KISS Policy – Keep It Short and Simple!

There is no perfect way to write your resume but these tips do work well in hand-holding through your profile creation journey.

# G - Interview Hygiene Checks

We discussed creating a powerful profile in the last capsule. Cracking an interview is a challenge for a lot of job seekers despite them being good candidates, and having impactful profiles and experiences too.

In my experience, there are some important elements that one needs to consider during the start to end of an interview process.

Let us begin with the Telephonic Interviews.

When you decide to apply for an opportunity, must-do homework includes researching about the organisation, their work and culture, the role, the money range, and travel time. Of course, you will not get work next to your home all the time but do consider your daily travel time, your stamina, and its possible impact on your productivity.

But study all of this before you apply. These questions should not be on your mind when you get an interview call or after a shortlist for that matter!

There is this one thing that you must never forget. Brand or Company Name, Profile and Pay are the three keys with which your job door opens.

You may not have all these keys to your access all the time. Remember, if you have two out of the three, you are good to go!

For beginners, please remember...
- Candidate A has received a very high CTC at the entry level.
- Candidate B has also received a good offer but less compared to A.

Both are entry-level postgraduates and their performance has been superb across the year. The organisation decides to appraise and promote both.

Keep in mind, that when you are promoted or even with getting senior at a company your responsibility increases and what is expected out of you also does.

But the monetary rise mainly depends on targeted v/s actual business for the year and many other elements which are way beyond only employee performance.

Besides, for every designation slab, there is a salary bracket or a range, most companies have pre-framed. I mean five employees of the same designation will not have the same salary of course but the range will obliviously be an aligned one.

So, coming back to Candidate A and B, while both did well, the incremental percentage will differ but end point will get them both in the pre-framed range.

This is to keep environmental harmony in the organisation.

Again, as you get senior, your work increases but the appraisal percentage may not increase at the same speed.

Hence the saturation points of entry level candidates who start with higher CTC's come earlier than others and the job switch frequencies as well.

This does not mean that you do not consider salary criteria but just make sure you keep in mind all of this.

Experienced candidates must do a complete study on the hike percentage and prepare to justify their quotes.

Being well-informed is half ready!

Telephonic interviews are extremely essential part of the selection process of many organisations, especially in the media fraternity since it is an extremely dynamic segment.

This makes it easy for prospective talent to be spontaneous, confident, and poised across forms of communication, over and above, he or she has the domain knowledge and the other criteria specified by the company.

Having applied for an opportunity, ensure you are well-read as most of the interviews come at short or no notices, be it – Telephonic or Face to Face.

For a pre-scheduled telephonic interview, be ready with your resume, all the job details along with the highlights of the organisation.

It is a good idea to keep with you a paper and pencil to make notes. If your telephonic interview is not a scheduled one, it is even more important for you to keep yourself in prepared mode!

If the telephonic interview is an unplanned one, request the caller for 30 seconds to get to a quiet place and organize stuff.

Introduce yourself. Always keep your voice modulation in tune with the conversation. A smile makes a big difference in a conversation, even on the phone.

Your voice reveals both your personality and your attitude towards the caller.

While you communicate, sound well-informed, talk with dignity and never sound all over the place

During the tele-talk, be calm and precise in your communication. Understand the question well before you answer.

Do not fidget with things or papers around. No shuffling papers in the background!

Your aim should be to communicate to the interviewer that you are the best candidate for the position, without sounding desperate, please! Let us now get to the Face-to-Face interviews.

Consider the Top 10 Hygiene Checks as you prepare:

- Greet the interviewer because it is one of the first impressions we leave on a panellist. Most of us feel that the interviewers are the ones sitting in the interview room either single or in a panel format.

Here is the thing; the one who opens the interview room door to call out our name for the interview also has a role to play in your selection process! The truth is we are so anxious now that it does not even strike us.

- Handshake with interview panellists - Once we are in the interview room, whether your initial gesture will be a head nod or a handshake needs to be an informed choice.

If the interview table speaks of the psychology of distance, we may choose to say good morning with a head nod. Else a handshake does it well. Here, in both cases, a pleasant smile with eye contact is necessary. Also, the handshake needs to be a professional one and not a fancy finger-palm touch!

- Seeking permission to have a seat - Once you are done with the greeting part, the interviewer will usually ask you to sit down. If not, take permission before you take your seat on the interviewee chair.
- Using the interview table: Once you are seated, remember that the interview table is the

interviewer's property and not yours. It is a good idea to not rest your hands or keep your belongings on the interview table.

- Introducing yourself - "Good morning, Sir / Ma'am (depending on the seniority), my name is Aditi". A lot of us tend to make errors here. Do remember that the interviewer has your resume with your name mentioned and you have already finished greeting them.

- Eye Contact –Make sure to have an eye contact with the panellist who has asked you the question, while answering until he or she is looking at you. Looking elsewhere or on the floor while you talk or while you are being spoken to is considered as inappropriate. This is crucial as it reflects on your confidence levels.

- Bluffing - There will be situations in an interview where you do not know the answer to a question asked. It is completely okay to politely accept that you are not aware of the answer. If you are not sure and wish to make a guess, word it that way. Bluffing or faking is a big no because often you are evaluated on the fact that whether you know that you do not know and how honestly you deal with it!

- Getting your body language right - While having an interview conversation if we tend to fidget with any stuff around, touch our face or hair often, or then shake our legs or tangle our hand fingers, and more of such stuff reflects signs of nervousness or that we are distracted. The key is to stay calm and maintain focus.

- Scripted Instances - A lot of us do not keep ready instances for value based and HRQ's. These questions are often asked to judge a candidate's personality or a specific behavioural skill. Here we are asked to give an instance of a dilemma handled or a decision taken or then a situation is given and the candidate is asked to opine or reflect.

- Do not miss it - Be ready with an interesting question to ask at the end of the interview. Often candidates are asked if they have any questions. You may ask about the organization, more about what is expected or something to that note depending on the shape your interview has taken during the conversation. If you realize you cannot do that, you may thank the interviewer for their time...

## H- The C-A-R Concept

We all go through a series of interviews in our job hunt phase, especially at the entry level positions. Let me share with you, a quick tip for a progressive interview.

The C-A-R concept can be applied to any situation of life. Here I am giving an extra brownie to our younger ones!

During an interview, when you are discussing your SWOT, it becomes non-negotiable to give examples to authenticate the points you speak about.

Telling the interviewer "I am the best" does not make him or her believe in you or dozens of candidates who may have said the same or similar.

Well! Story telling is not confined to media alone! It is universal. Yes, your narrative will depend on your resume and profile. So, ensure that you have:

- Shaped up a well aligned resume with supportive documents to your mentions.
- Read up about the company, the role and your resume to be in sync with it.
- You know your resume as much as your resume knows you.
- Are prepared for the interview.

Ready? Come On! Let's GET SET GO...

Here, make sure that you use, what I call as the

C-A-R Concept... And I will tell you what it means.

|| Context || Action || Result ||

Interviewer: Tell me something about your strengths

Interviewee: I am proactive and possess leadership skills

Here is an example of how you can apply the CAR Concept to your answer to make it more real-time.

C – Context (Background information of situation)

Interviewee: During my MBA, I pursued a marketing internship with XYZ. We were five interns from different colleges. Our role was to reach out to brands to find the relevant point of contact and line up appointments for the director to present the business pitch.

It was the last week of the month and as a team of interns, we were needed to reach a target of 100, which meant 20 per head. On day 3 of the week, one of the interns fell ill and was advised bed rest.

Another intern was thinking of withdrawing from the internship as she could not handle the pressure building up. That left us with 3 interns with the same target.

A – Action (Your contribution)

Interviewee: It was a difficult situation as I too was an intern. But I decided that I would give it my best shot. First, I spoke to the intern who was breaking down and cheered her to team up to with the best possible. Next, I took in confidence the other two interns and convinced them that we can and shall pull it through, only that instead of 100% we will shell out 120% of effort each for the next 3-4 days.

I also told them that the intern who was breaking down has somehow agreed to try her best but she may fall weak and we may need to double up.

With a coffee and cheers, we started our mission, planned our daily connect points with buffers, and waited back late on the remaining days of the week to cut it through.

R – Result (What did your action make happen?)

Interviewee: On the last day of the week, our reporting was at 6.30pm and I, along with the team of three interns managed to present them a report of 100!

Though I penned an example of MBA life to explain the CAR Concept, this a utility tool that can be applied across situations by all age groups to align to various circumstances on a positive strike rate.

# I - Unfolding Stakeholder Harmony

In the world of business, be it a fresher or an experienced professional, the one highest-rated skill that stands out is the art of stakeholder relations, as it forms the basis of professional success.

Imagine a weave where each thread represents a stakeholder, from loyal customers to dedicated employees, vigilant investors, and benevolent community members.

The adept steward of stakeholder relations skilfully navigates this intricate landscape, threading communications and nurturing the dance of engagement, every step is a symphony of connections, from one-on-one meetings to town hall gatherings.

Through dialogue, insights are captured, concerns are ironed out, and visions are shared, laying the foundations for collaborations

But let us not forget the delicate art of conflict resolution, where skilled practitioners sync in equilibrium and adaptability by forging pathways to reconciliation, and harmony and mutual benefit.

Yet, in this ever-evolving space of stakeholder relations, stagnation finds no solace and embraces the ethos of continuous improvement, refining their craft with each passing day.

In the theatre of a progressive endeavour, the spotlight shines brightly upon the virtuoso of stakeholder relations.

With a flourish of finesse, let us seek ten touch points to understand and identify our stakeholders well enough that every voice is heard and finds a place in the tapestry of progress:

- Which tasks does your stakeholder dread doing? Example: Asking the board for more money for her project.
- What confuses your stakeholder as it relates to your project?
  Example: My stakeholder does not understand that my questions are only to seek clarity for concluding towards informed choices.
- What kind of people does your stakeholder seek out for advice? Example: My stakeholder usually seeks out to his good friend from purchasing.
- What is your stakeholder's career dream? Example: Starting a consulting firm.
- What is your stakeholder's life dream? Example: My stakeholder wishes he could retire early.
- What makes your stakeholder feel embarrassed or self-conscious? Example: Not being able to answer questions asked.

- What competes for your stakeholder's attention?

    Example: A strategic implementation.

- What are your stakeholder's concerns as it relates to your cooperation? Example: They will be held responsible for decisions they did not make or and do not agree with.
- How does your stakeholder want to be perceived? Example: As an employee who always delivers on his promises.
- What kind of rewards does your stakeholder prefer? Example: Monetary and non-monetary.

I would suggest you plot your premise through the funnel of these nuggets to optimize its value-ad.

## J - Your Transfer-ables'

In Dr. Swati Lodha's November 2022 release, '360 Degree Excellence', she beautifully narrated the need to be a transfer learner and its essence in mapping up with the P- pods of human life.

Transfer Learner essentially entails switching the P2P roles, for instance - student to work-life and further on which involves tuning back and forth and at times by the clock.

This requires skills in alignment. Hence need for having various skills is crucial to accomplish our desired goals across walks of life. Skills are a must-have, be it work life, study life or personal life.

I have heard many say "I am a beginner; I do not have any skill. They will not select me for the job." For that matter, even senior professionals are not excluded from this.

Well, skills are transferable! - Yes, they are! They are called transferable skills. By this I mean, that the skills that we acquire while pursuing any activity during our routines - employment, projects, voluntary work, hobbies, or sports can be applied at a later stage in newer situations, meaning they can be transferred.

Some of the popular transferable skills include – self management, communication, trouble shooting, time management, and being proactive...

Let us now look at the transferable skills cycle:

- Skill Acquisition: A skill acquired through the routine activity performed. For example: In a group project in college, we learn team work, time management and troubleshooting issues.
- Skill Progression: The acquired skill is identified and further developed to be able to put it to use ahead. It could be in the form of a professional training or doing more of such activities to polish up the skill.
- Skill Match: While applying for a job role, I read the job descriptions and specifications carefully, shaped up my resume accordingly as I now know that I have the said skill sets.

Then I decide and act on it - Apply, Prep Up and Step Up!

- Skill Transfer: I will now apply the skills at my work, that is for the new situation

Pro-Tip: Reflect and Record all the transferable skills you identify into your log book because you will eventually realise that skill transfer is again a journey and not a destination. So be the STAR!

S-Situation - Secured my placement with X Company, working as a junior

T-Task - Assigned to work on the start-upand assisted the department head in achieving departmental targets and standards.

A-Action - Was responsible for... from start through to finish. Carried out tests and recorded results.... Implemented new system......

R-Results - Developed strong communication skills in liaising with key personnel at weekly progress meetings. Improved my problem-solving skills through researching possible solutions, analysing options, and identifying optimum solutions.

Developed project management skills by planning work, setting deadlines, managing workload, prioritising daily tasks, and achieving goals

This was a generic example to demonstrate the application of the tool. Feed in your premise of the situation and adapt the tool for a progressive outcome.

# K - Emma's Mid-Career Era

Once upon a time, in the city of Metropolis, there lived a young professional named Emma. Emma started her career with passion and determination, eager to climb the corporate ladder and make a meaningful impact in her field of marketing.

As years went by, Emma found herself at a mid-career crossroads. She had achieved moderate success but felt a growing sense of stagnation and uncertainty about her future. Reflecting on her journey so far, Emma realized she needed to reassess her goals.

Firstly, she decided to sharpen her skills. She enrolled in advanced marketing courses and attended workshops on digital trends and analytics. Emma knew that staying relevant in her field meant continuously learning and adapting to new technologies and consumer behaviour.

Secondly, Emma focused on expanding her professional network. She joined industry associations, attended conferences, and actively engaged in online communities. Through networking, she not only gained valuable insights but also discovered new career opportunities and collaborations.

Thirdly, Emma prioritized her brand. She revamped her LinkedIn profile, started writing articles on marketing strategies, and spoke at local meet-ups. Establishing herself as a thought leader not only boosted her credibility but also opened doors to speaking engagements and consulting opportunities.

However, amidst all these efforts, Emma realized the importance of work-life integration. She started dedicating time to hobbies she loved, such as painting and hiking. These activities not only refreshed her mind but also provided new perspectives that she could apply to her work.

One day, Emma received a surprising offer from a prestigious marketing firm. They were impressed by her skills, network, and personal brand. The offer came with a significant promotion and the opportunity to lead a team of talented marketers. Emma accepted the offer, excited for the new challenges ahead.

As she settled into her new role, Emma reflected on her journey through the mid-career phase. The essentials–continuous learning, networking, building a personal brand, and maintaining work-life alignment – had been crucial in shaping her success. She knew that the lessons learned during this phase would guide her towards achieving even greater milestones in her career.

And so, Emma's story serves as a reminder to all mid-career professionals to invest in these essentials, embrace new challenges, and never stop striving for growth and fulfilment in their career journey.

Quick Tips from Emma's journey:

Tip: Stay updated with industry trends and acquire new skills relevant to your field.

Example: Attend conferences like the Tech Summit to learn about the latest advancements in AI and machine learning, or enrol in online courses like Coursera's Digital Marketing Specialization to enhance your skills in digital marketing.

Tip: Actively participate in industry events, join professional associations, and maintain meaningful connections.

Example: Regularly attend meet-ups organized by the Marketing Association and engage with peers on LinkedIn to expand your network. For instance, connecting with speakers after a conference session can lead to valuable collaborations or job opportunities.

Tip: Take on leadership roles in projects or mentor junior colleagues to enhance your leadership abilities.

Example: Volunteer to lead cross-functional teams on major projects within your company, such as heading the annual marketing campaign. Alternatively, mentor junior marketers on best practices in campaign strategy, leveraging your expertise and fostering a supportive team culture.

Tip: Establish yourself as a thought leader by sharing insights and showcasing your expertise.

Example: Start a blog where you discuss emerging trends in marketing strategies or contribute articles to industry publications like Marketing Profs. Additionally, actively participate in panel discussions at industry conferences to demonstrate your knowledge and thought leadership.

Tip: Prioritize self-care and set boundaries to avoid burnout.

Example: Dedicate time to hobbies or activities that bring you joy and relaxation, such as yoga or painting. Set aside non-work hours for family and friends to recharge and maintain a healthy work-life balance.

Tip: Stay agile and open to new opportunities or career shifts.

Example: Consider taking on a new role or exploring a different industry segment that aligns with your skills and interests. For instance, transitioning from traditional marketing to digital marketing roles can provide fresh challenges and opportunities for growth.

Tip: Assess Transferable Skills and Knowledge.

Example: If you are transitioning from finance to marketing, skills in data analysis and strategic planning are transferable. Highlight these skills on your resume and during interviews to demonstrate their relevance.

Tip: Stay Resilient and Open to Feedback.

Example: Seek feedback from peers, mentors, or hiring managers during the transition process. Use constructive criticism to refine your approach and adapt as needed.

Finally... Be Patient and Persistent because switching domains may take time and perseverance. Keep applying for relevant positions, networking, and improving your skills.

Stay committed to your goal and celebrate small achievements along the way.

We all, at some point in time, have stepped or will step into Emma's shoes, reasons may be different. By focusing on these tips, professionals in their mid-career eras can navigate challenges, seize growth opportunities, and continue advancing towards fulfilling and successful career trajectories.

# Segment III –A:
## Student Community Special

# A - Unlocking Academic Excellence

Achieving academic success in college is not just about attending lectures and memorizing textbooks; it requires a strategic approach to learning and mastering various skills. From effective study habits to managing time efficiently and handling exam stress, here is a comprehensive guide to help you excel in your academic journey.

Developing effective study habits lays the foundation for academic achievement. Here are some proven strategies:

- Create a Dedicated Study Space: Designate a quiet, well-lit area specifically for studying. Ensure it is free from distractions like mobiles or tablets and the like.
- Use Active Learning Techniques: Instead of passively reading, engage actively with the material. Summarize chapters in your own words, create concept maps, or teach the content to a study partner.
- Practice Regularly: Schedule consistent study sessions rather than cramming. Spacing out your study sessions over time enhances retention.
- Utilize Multiple Resources: Combine textbooks with online resources, videos, and

supplementary materials to gain a deeper understanding of the subject matter.
- Dealing with Exam Stress: Exams can be stressful, but with proper preparation and stress management techniques, you can navigate them confidently.
- Start Early: Begin studying well in advance to avoid cramming. Review class notes regularly and create study guides.
- Practice Past Exams: Familiarize yourself with the exam format and types of questions asked. Practice under timed conditions to simulate exam pressure.
- Practice Relaxation Techniques: Deep breathing, mindfulness, or physical exercise can help alleviate stress and improve focus.
- Get Adequate Rest: Prioritize sleep during exam periods. A well-rested mind performs better and retains information more effectively.

Few lucrative academic writing tips:
- Clear and effective communication through writing is essential for academic success.
- Understand the Assignment: Carefully read the assignment prompt and clarify any doubts with your professor.

- Plan and Outline: Before writing, outline your ideas and structure your paper logically. This helps in organizing thoughts and arguments.
- Use Clear and Concise Language: Write in a formal tone and avoid jargon unless necessary. Be succinct and articulate your points effectively.
- Revise and Edit: Proofread your work for grammar, punctuation, and coherence. Consider seeking feedback from peers or tutors for constructive criticism.
- By implementing these study tips and techniques, you can enhance your learning experience, manage your time effectively, alleviate exam stress, and refine your academic writing skills.

Remember, academic success is not just about grades but also about developing lifelong learning habits that will serve you well beyond college. Embrace these strategies, adapt them to your needs, and watch your academic journey flourish, and find its best version.

# B - Top Skill Spots for a Lucrative Profession

Being in training management and having interacted with academicians, recruiters, and functional heads across corporate entities over the years, I have learnt and analysed with deep thought that there are six major skills evaluated during a hiring process.

From inducting an aspirant into a PG program or then into a selection process for career opportunities, the tragedy is that despite everything, most aspirants struggle with more than one of these skills at any point in time. In this piece, I will spell out crucial key spots.

Communication: You have read my previous capsule on Top 10 Tools for High Impact Communication and by now you know that it is one of the most crucial skills needed for even the simplest of conversations. Coming to the selection process across levels - communication is the default key!

Trust me, I have seen a lot of senior people unable to complete the cycle of communication without even realizing it. With entry level candidates the candidates, the challenge is slightly different.

Here is the thing.

Communication is not English. It is about being crisp and effective while we talk. Speak in a way that your message, be it oral or written - is clearly understood by the receiver. To achieve this situation, however good you may be, some basic self-help is a must.

Read, Read, and Read - Pick up a book of your choice - fiction or non-fiction or then something related to the work domain you want to opt for.

When you are reading, keep a dictionary, paper, and a pen handy. Write the new words you come across, understand their meanings and the reference to the context in which they are used and gradually adapt the words in your conversation.

Of course, you may choose to seek professional help based on your present state.

Pro - Tip: Reading improves vocabulary and ability to articulate which is very important to be able to communicate effectively.

Yesterday I was chatting to a friend's son who is in his twenties, discussing his plans. He is in his final year of graduation and was trying to connect the dots to taking up higher studies after his final year.

His academics through schooling and graduation college was not all that great so I told him to buck up in the final at least because that may act as an obstacle later.

I told him to figure out two things:
- The colleges and programs on his wish list.
- Sources to connect and reach out to the concerned people.

Networking and Resourcefulness: This is a primary criterion for both, higher study, and work life. Network is Net Worth!

Majority of the best resources are available to you through your network, from classmates to mentors, colleagues to seniors and stakeholders at large.

Pro - Tip: Take small initiatives to meet new people. Whether you are studying, on a job hunt or at your workplace.

From classrooms to conferences, seminars, and events... unfold each opportunity.

A platform like LinkedIn helps big time in connecting with people across hierarchies, domains, and locations.

Your Top Must Haves Include:

- Business Acumen or Industry Understanding: In any selection process the evaluator or a recruiter is always keen to know if you as a candidate or an aspirant have some know - how of the chosen field or profession.

    For example: They will not ask you questions like defining money or the importance of PR. What they would like to know is how aware you are about business environments in general and whether you carry a basic understanding of the preferred domain. And yes, your reasons for choosing what you have chosen.

Pro - Tip: To cover this point with efficiency, Reading and Networking is the spot you need to capitalize on.

- Digital Literacy, Creative and MIS Tools: Super utilities like Sheets, Docs, Slides, Canva, Forms and similar utilities required across job functions and hence extremely important to be hands-on with.

Pro- Tip: Take professional training on these online or offline, whatever works for you but do it for sure. And yes, figure out avenues to stay connected with what you have learnt.

- Aptitude and Attitude: When an organization looks at hiring a candidate, they want to first check on the reasoning abilities of the person.
- Are you a problem solver in approach?
- Can you think on your feet or not?
- Are you a culture fit by mindset or not?

And most importantly, your domain knowledge and whether you can transfer that domain knowledge into essential skills needed for the work role.

Pro-Tip: Let us be realistic.

Each person is unique and has skills and abilities. At times these skill sets may be aligned by God's gift. But that is rare a case to well sync with.

Developing them is the need of the hour most of the times

Fact: Knowledge, Skills, Aptitude and Attitude hold equal weightage as employability quotients.

Opportunities for experiential impact also play big time in developing your profile

- Network and Branding: Not every one of us is an influencer, so you may feel why networking and personal branding are needed. Well. The truth is social listening is as important for marketers as for talent hunting. Organizations do consider the social media presence of potential hires. This is to get a feel of what kind of stuff the candidate talks or writes about, his or her opinions about various occurrences and what he or she is followed for.

Pro -Tip: Read up and start writing about topics related to your domain. That is how you will get known for a particular topic. The best-suited platforms for this are ones like LinkedIn.

Finally, your resume. We have discussed it in detail in my previous capsule.

Higher Education plays a huge role in nurturing your candidature with a holistic perspective. Of course, your complete commitment towards your progress is non-negotiable, whatever the direction you pick!

# C - Work and Vocals go hand-in-hand

If you are someone who feels that language is your weakness, you will in all probability have a jitter of not being able to crack interviews because your communication is not mapping up.

Of course, one cannot deny that the English language is the need of the hour in a lot of places.

However, First things First.

So, communication exactly?

Here is the thing.

Communication is about speaking, writing, or expressing its purpose.

The purpose here is the interview.

In my experience, the five aspects of communication that matter during an interview are:

Vocabulary is not about knowing fancy words. When you use jargons during an interview that becomes the first indication of being at a cross. Having a good vocabulary means that you know and can use the appropriate words to articulate and communicate what you need to convey, maybe your thoughts or ideas or the answers to what you have been asked. This means that you do not need random vocabulary but rather specifics that suit the purpose or are related to the situation.

Pro- Tip: Always keep a pocket dictionary at hand. Identify five new words every day with their meaning and try to utilize them in your routine conversations. I do it even today - interview or no interview.

Fluency: You may think, "Oh! That someone is so fluent and quick when they are speaking". The truth is fluency is not speed. Fluency here is about being able to communicate with ease and be understood with the same ease by the listener with expressions you lent out during the conversation.

Pro - Tip: Stand in front of the mirror and speak loud and clear at a normal pace with appropriate expression or seek help from a friend who can give you constructive feedback.

Practice: While they say, 'Practice Makes Man Perfect,' rehearsing more does not always guarantee success.

Besides, the possibilities of forgetting parrot work are always higher. So best is to keep it simple.

No one at an interview expects you to rote memorize your intro in a creative way and puke.

What is needed is your ability to transfer your opinion or experience related to what has been asked of you.

Pro - Tip: List down relevant experiences which you can use during an interview depending on the question that comes your way. This will also allow you to sink in the flow.

For instance: What is the biggest challenge you faced?

Your answer should include:
- What happened?
- Consequences...
- How I got affected?
- How did I bounce back?

Non-Verbal Cues: Body language and expressions play a very important role in an interview. For instance:

Posture: A backward lean shows resistance anda forward lean shows over-flown towards the other
- Eye contact: increases trust element.
- Handshake reveals belief in yourself.

Here reference to context changes on both sides of the table.

Listening is one of the most important communication skills. While you listen to what is being told or asked because it helps you respond better, it is necessary to be observant as well.

Pro - Tip: Impactful orators always listen attentively to make their response powerful.

There is this one skill I learnt from one of the books I read some time back. It is 'Referencing'.

Here you use one of the elements of your current environment to explain with a turnaround, any of the things asked.

It is about converting a weakness into an opportunity by using relevant reference to context.

For example - What is your weakness?

Say vulnerability, you had either read about courage somewhere or then just picked on reverse gear.

You can mention vulnerability by saying, "One must walk through vulnerability to reach courage."

The message you are giving out will be that you are someone who accepts what it is, is observant, and knows how to mould toward progress.

## D – Seven Step Guide to Choosing your MBA Program

Are you considering pursuing your post-graduation but feeling overwhelmed by the myriads of options available?

Choosing the right business school can be a daunting task, but fear not! Here is a Seven Step Guide with some food for thought which will help you navigate through your journey.

- Goal Setting: Before diving into the sea post-graduation, take some time to reflect on your career aspirations and what you hope to gain from it. Are you looking to advance in your current field, pivot to a new industry, or start your own business? Clarifying your goals will help you narrow down your options and find a program that aligns with your objectives.

- Credibility: Ensure that the business schools you are considering are accredited by reputable accrediting bodies to ensure that the program meets certain quality standards and will be recognized by employers. Considering international degrees from reputed universities can also be a point. Non-negotiable here is to look for rankings, alumni success stories, and employer perceptions. But that is not all. The academic fabric needs to be one of the major factors to look at.

- Curriculum and Specializations: Evaluate the curriculum of the programs to see if it offers the courses and specializations that align with your interests and career goals. Some programs may have a focus on entrepreneurship, finance, marketing, or other areas. Choose a program that offers a curriculum tailored to your needs. Also, before doing so, evaluate your interest to the "reals" not the "reels". By this I mean your skills.

My interest lies in making tea, but I am a skilled at making coffee!

I will discuss the crucial skills for progressions in HR, Marketing, Media and Finance domains in the next capsule.

- Faculty and Resources: Research the faculty members of the program to ensure they are experts in their fields and have relevant industry experience. Look at skill-based programs because skills are what your potential recruiter looks at. Additionally, consider the resources available to students, such as career services, networking opportunities, and an exhaustive corporate interface. A supportive and resource-rich environment can greatly enhance your post-graduation experience and help you achieve your goals.

- Location and Network: Consider the location of the business school and its proximity to potential employers and industry hubs. For instance, a school located in a major city or business centre may offer more networking opportunities and access to internships and job opportunities. Also do consider the alumni network of each school and the strength of its connections in your desired industry.

- Cost and Financial Aid: MBA programs can be a significant financial investment, so it is important to consider the cost of tuition, fees, and living expenses. Research scholarship opportunities, financial aid options, and potential return on investment to ensure that you are making a wise financial decision.

- Visit and Connect: Whenever possible, visit the campuses of the school you are considering and attend information sessions or open houses. This will give you a feel of the culture, facilities, and community. It is a good idea to reach out to current students and alumni to get their insights and perspectives on the program.

The training content, pedagogy, trainers, and corporate engagement opportunities make the key to the lock. While the look and feel of the college may just be normal, look at considering what matters most.

Choosing the right program is a crucial step in advancing your career and achieving your professional goals.

By considering these factors and doing your due diligence, you can find the perfect business school that will set you on the path to success.

# E- Setting your base for Finance, Marketing and Human Resource Functions

Exploring Opportunities in Finance: In today's fast-paced financial world, success is not just about crunching numbers; it is about mastering a diverse set of skills that go beyond traditional finance expertise.

Honing these top five skills can set you on the path to a thriving career in finance.

- Communication Skills: Effective communication is essential for building relationships, presenting findings, and influencing decisions in finance. Whether it is crafting a compelling investment pitch or explaining financial concepts to clients, strong communication skills are vital. For instance, an investment banker must communicate complex financial information clearly and persuasively to clients to secure deals and build trust.

- Analytical Thinking: The ability to analyze complex data sets and draw meaningful insights is crucial in finance. Employers seek candidates who can interpret financial statements, assess investment opportunities, and identify trends in the market. For example, a financial analyst might use analytical thinking to evaluate the performance of a company by analysing its cash flow, profitability ratios, and market trends to make informed investment recommendations.

- Adaptability: The finance industry is constantly evolving, driven by technological advancements, regulatory changes, and shifting market dynamics. Professionals need to be adaptable and embrace change to stay ahead of the curve. This could mean learning new software tools, staying updated on industry trends, or adapting investment strategies to changing market conditions. For instance, a financial planner may need to adapt their advice to clients based on changes in tax laws or economic conditions.

- Risk Management: Finance is by default bonded to risk, and a finance aspirant must be adept at assessing, mitigating, and managing risks effectively. This involves understanding various risk factors, such as market volatility, credit risk, and regulatory changes, and implementing strategies to minimize their impact. A risk manager, like one might need to develop support strategies to protect against market fluctuations

- Ethical Decision-Making: Integrity and ethical conduct are non-negotiable in finance, where trust and credibility are paramount. For example, a compliance officer plays a crucial role in ensuring that a company's operations comply with legal and regulatory requirements, safeguarding its reputation and integrity.

Of course, every organization will have their protocols for hiring fresher's or even when they seek experienced potentials, honing these bare minima of essentials in finance, you can seek opportunities in the following verticals.

From traditional roles in investment banking and accounting to emerging fields like fintech and sustainable finance, the finance industry offers a multitude of paths for professionals to pursue their passions and carve out rewarding careers.

Yes, it is a good idea to remember that, between your goal and you, their lies a journey to travel.

- Investment Banking: is known for its fast-paced environment and high-stake deals, investment banking offers unparalleled opportunities for those with a knack for financial analysis, strategic thinking, and relationship-building.
- Corporate Finance: In some organizations, in-house finance teams are responsible for managing the company's finances, analysing investments, and optimizing capital structure. Careers in corporate finance offer exposure to a wide range of responsibilities, including

financial planning and analysis, treasury management, and risk assessment.

- Asset Management: Asset managers oversee investment portfolios on behalf of individuals, institutions, and funds, aiming to maximize returns while managing risk. These opportunities involve researching investment opportunities, constructing portfolios, and implementing investment strategies tailored to clients' objectives.
- Financial Technology (Fintech): The intersection of finance and technology has given rise to the booming field of fintech, revolutionizing how financial services are delivered and consumed.
- Risk Management and Compliance: In an increasingly complex regulatory environment, risk management and compliance have become critical functions within financial institutions.

While these were some of the prominent opportunities one can look at, the finance industry offers a vast array of options suited to individuals with diverse interests, skills, and aspirations.

If you are a beginner, ensure having polished up on your financial modelling skills, understanding and interpreting financial statements, tools like excel or python, data skills and a conceptual understanding of the terminologies used, what and how they imply, couple of job simulations and an internship. Its non-negotiable to deep dive into the domain beyond academics if you are someone looking at a sustainable career, irrespective of the domain.

A periodic up-skill holds equal importance for experienced professionals as well. Hope these nuggets help you navigate through your journey towards a lucrative career in the finance domain.

The Marketing Nuggets:

If you are interested in pursuing a career in marketing, honing these top five skills is essential for success in this ever-evolving field.

First and foremost, Strategic Thinking is the cornerstone of effective marketing. This involves analysing data, understanding market trends via research and forecasting, and identifying opportunities to reach target audiences. For instance, developing a comprehensive marketing plan that aligns with business objectives and leverages consumer insights to drive growth.

Understanding data and analytics is also fundamental for making informed decisions and optimizing marketing strategies. Analytical Skills come into play when analysing sales data for a product, identifying which marketing strategies have been most effective in driving sales, and suggesting adjustments to future marketing campaigns based on your findings.

Creativity in marketing involves the ability to generate unique ideas, concepts, and strategies to attract and engage customers. Creating an attention-grabbing advertising campaign that uses humour, storytelling, or visually striking imagery to connect with the target audience is a prime example. This skill allows marketers to leave a memorable impression on consumers.

Communication and Collaboration are keys to building strong relationships with cross-functional teams, customers, colleagues, and stakeholders. Clear and compelling communication is essential for conveying brand messages and driving engagement, whether it is crafting persuasive messages, delivering impactful presentations, or engaging with followers on social media.

Lastly, Adaptability and Time Management skills are crucial for progress in a constantly evolving landscape. Being able to pivot quickly, embrace change, and innovate in response to shifting market dynamics is essential. Additionally, strong time management skills are essential for staying organized and prioritizing tasks effectively.

In the Marketing space, you can seek opportunities in Brand, Product or Services Marketing, both traditional and digital.

The 'H' and 'R' of HR (Human Resources): The HR field offers lucrative career paths for individuals with diverse skill sets. From recruitment to talent acquisition, employee relations to learning and development, and compensation and benefits to HR strategy, the possibilities are endless.

For entry-level positions, you can start with talent acquisition (TA), which involves sourcing, screening, and hiring top-tier talent. Or, you can explore learning and developmentto empower teams through continuous growth and skill development. If you have a knack for resolving conflicts and fostering a positive work culture, employee relations might be the right fit for you. As you gain experience and expertise you can look at HR Business Partnership roles and much more!

# F -Media and Content Mantras

Do you like communicating with people, giving them information about occurrences and happenings around them? About a new movie coming up or about a new shampoo launch? About essentials during a crisis? Yes?

Then Media is a profession you can consider. To help you understand Media broadly, let me first tell you about the eight simple steps of communication.

- Observe the behaviour of your audiences, how they interact, how they think and feel and what are their community values and interests.
- Listening takes off all the development guess works. One of the best ways to do this is to add social media intelligence to your network to uncover the key conversations by your audiences about any given topic.
- Identify key Influencers on the topic, people and communities who are influential to thought process and look at associating with them.
- Internalize what you have gathered from observations and listening to develop meaningful content to work on.

- Share the knowledge with different departments of your organization to collate the blanks in the content you have gathered.
- Process the information from a 360-degree perspective.
- Participate; open communication is a good source to create a peer-to-peer approach.
- Feedback, contributes to making information more relevant and concise for the desired audiences.

To summarise, media about communicating strategically at the right time, to the right people, a precise message through the appropriate communication tool.

PR, Public Relations, one of the key power packed media tools comes with as much excitement as much of thought and smart work. Like Advertising, PR also follows an AIDA phase. Awareness before an occurrence, during occurrence and after the occurrence, for a planned format activity.

As a PR person your role is diverse. Say you are doing PR for the brand - Sunsilk. Your 1st task at hand will be to understand the brand, it is audiences and its competition. Staying tuned to your brand and competitive updates is crucial. That will aid your PR moves for Sunsilk.

Next you will need to identify, ideate, and execute PR-able opportunities for your brand. For example, considering female audiences for Sunsilk, you could plan online or offline engagements for occasions like Women's Day and Mother's Day.

In summary, there are these seasonal and occasional tools for interacting with audiences.

As a business opportunity, you will plan on Sunsilk associating with a Filmfare Awards or any televised / non televised event. You could plan for Sunsilk endorsing itself within a movie or a show just like Nescafe in Sanjivini - 2 on Hotstar. This means you are creating media visibility for your brand, which is again very necessary.

Public Relations also calls for back-end roles like media relations, planning and positioning, writing and content creation, and reputation management. PR is like parenting a brand through all the odds and evens of its life cycle.

Public Relations as an industry is an investment of time, money for brand communications that leads to credibility and relationship building. It is critical to any brand that needs media exposure, requires to sway consumer opinion, and maintain good will.

Modern - age PR demands an integrated, well planned and a multi-channel approach that aids in amplifying the brand message to audiences. Hence PR one of the strongest business support tools.

Getting on to Advertising...

When you think of a brand, what comes to your mind? L'Oreal? Adidas? Netflix? Cadbury?

These companies have spent millions of rupees and thousands of hours of hard work for their names to pop into our heads.

That is what advertising is all about!

There have been a lot of prominent marketing models and one of them being the 4P's - product, price, place, and promotions. The 4P's form the base of the strategy you create to get your brand message to your audiences - Right audiences, Right message, Right time, High on ROI and Low on cost.

A great question would be, "How do I get the best from my brand?"

A lot has changed in the world of advertising in the last decade. But one thing remains the same - A great idea, executed brilliantly can change the fortune of your brand.

Brands need their messages to reach the audiences appropriately, which will ultimately help their revenue streams grow.

There are agencies in multiples working on brand promotions and are in constant search of fresh talent and perspectives to contribute to the communication business in various capacities.

There are 360-degree advertising agencies which function as full-service agencies, with everything under one roof type. Also, there are independent media, creative, digital marketing, outdoor, events and pr agencies which caters to the specific services for brands.

Let us broadly understand the prominent job roles in an advertising agency:

Say for instance, Mr. A is the brand manager at KFC and has been asked to plan out for a 10% increase in revenues this financial year. He is to look out for an advertising agency to aid in achieving his business goal.

Mr. A will share the business brief and invite a shortlisted six best-suited advertising agencies for a pitch plan of how they will make the business goal a success.

The first to encounter Mr. A is the client servicing or account management team of the advertising agency.

- The Account Management (Client / Brand Services) team has two major roles including identifying and pitching new business for the agency and handling the advertising cycle for the brands on board.

This means you as a client servicing executive will handle the entire communication and coordination with the brand (in this case Mr. A) and with different teams within your agency to get the work done as per the client's brief.

- Planning / Strategy - Based on the brief received from the client, this team is responsible for creating the pitch deck and brand plan for the client/brand. This means you as a strategist will research, ideate, number crunch and come up with a plan to match the business goal of the brand.

You will also contribute to the execution bit, monitor progress and work on alternative strategies if the progress is not as desired.

- Creative Solutions - As a creative team member you will be involved in copywriting. Here you will ideate captions for different ad formats and churn out creative and impactful marketing copies for the brand keeping in mind the plan created by the strategy team to meet the business goal of the brand. The art team or visualiser's will work on the look, feel and aesthetics of the promotion materials - logos, creative's, banners, posters etc. This function works hand in hand with the strategy.

- Media Services - As a media planner, you will work hand in hand with the strategy team to identify and plan the media vehicles on which the brand needs to be promoted and the commercials involved. This means you suggest an action on whether KFC should advertise on TV / Print / Radio / Outdoor or Digital along with duration, tenure, frequency, and money.

- Integrated Services - The team mainly looks at opportunities for the brand to be integrated into different short and long-story formats. In this case, you will pitch KFC to different TV or Web Shows, Films or Events.

The role calls for different avenues to increase brand awareness and reinforcement.

Ad films and corporate films play a huge role in the advertising of a brand.

At times the advertising agency has its inbuilt production team or they look at outsourcing the project to a production house. The production house works on producing and packaging the end-to-end TVC keeping the client and strategy brief as a base.

It is all about the Business of Content... I call it Content Mantras!

Creating Marketable Content and Being Able to Market it is one of the Key Mantras of the Media and Communication Industry'.

A sector that revolves around the creation, marketing, and distribution of content across mediums like TV, Radio, Films, Digital, OTT to name the main ones.

Today, the entire world is talking about content. We get to hear this so very often and say it even more – "The content was not so good" or then , "The story rocked the show".

What is rocking or poor about content?

It is simple, if I as a consumer feels it worthy to read, hear, or see the content, subscribe, or buy a product or service after seeing, reading, or listening to the piece of communication, it is good and if not, it makes no meaning.

"If Consumer is the King, Your Content needs to be the Queen". Only then can you get them married!

Today I will share a few basic yet crucial key points to assist you in keeping your consumer hooked to your content.

- Begin with the end in mind

Why are you doing what you are doing? How do you want your audience to feel? What you want them to think? How do you want them to react after viewing what you show them? What is the purpose of your activity? What are you telling them what you are?

Do you want them to go to your website, make them aware of your product, download your app, subscribe to your service, watch your show, laugh, cry, or buy or then something else?

It is important to have answers to all these questions before you put across the communication you desire to. If you do not have the answers to these basic questions, there are huge chances of your communication not coming across the way it needs to.

- Identify the features

It is a good idea to ask your self-questions like, why will my audience listen to me? Why will they watch my show? Why will they consume my product or subscribe to my service? What is the value they need to see in it? How am I different or better than others in my business?

The more your communication stands crisp and clear, the better chances of you getting a response.

The more relate-able your content is, the better chances of your audience giving you a desired reaction. In summary, a brag sheet about your product or service helps big time in making precise communications about your brand or story.

- Who are you talking to?

Whom are you conversing with? What is important for them? What will drive them? Who are they?

For instance, the Colgate toothpaste commercial communicates to two types of audiences, the first one being P -To - P, (Parent to Parent), where a mother holding her toddler in her arms and saying, "mein apne bacche ke liye sirf Colgate pe hi bharosa karti hoon."

The other one is a C-To-C, (Child to Child), where a mother who is also a dentist is explaining the essence of strong teeth to a bunch of nursery school kids and one of the kids picks up the Colgate tooth paste pack saying, "my teeth strongest."

Sketch your consumer's bio or persona in your mind. Give them a name, a face and pen down about them, 'a day in the life of' to know about them and where does the need of your products and services feature in their day and how.

It is also important to know what do they want - products, services, value, or something else.

It is crucial to be sure of where does your communication fit in, in to your consumers day. Only then you will know what and how to communicate.

- Well started is half done!

This is a very popular phrase, heard by us multiple times at various occasions. The headline is your start. The first key role of your headline is to grab the attention of Mr. King, your consumer.

The headline should create curiosity in the mind of your audience in a way that they would desire to know more about what is in there.

They should want to listen to your story till the end or at least maximum possible. Be it a show, an ad, or an email.

A lot of times headlines or synopsis or 'about me' targeting concerns or aspirations of your audience helps in it being impactful.

If you are telling a story of something your consumer is living with or in, he / she will relate with it better and want to listen to you more.

A recent show on Netflix, 'Mumbai Begums' has ideated a great way of creating curiosity in the female audience's mind about the story just by the way they have written a short synopsis.

'It is a story of five ambitious women from different walks of life figuring their dreams, desires, and disappointments through their journeys'.

A short about me is enough for female masses consuming Netflix to watch the show.

If your headline or title can address a concern of its audience, it increases the probability of the consumer identifying with your communication and the chances of him / her staying on-board gets higher.

An effective piece here, the Sensodyne toothpaste ad. The communication starts with a lady biting a piece of candy ice cream and giving a deep expression of "daanton mein zhanghanahat" and discomfort.

The viewers easily identify their ice cream eating experiences and relate to the expressions and concerns.

Your start or headline can either create the moment of truth for your consumer or even become a reason to kill it.

- Avoid too many layers

Span of attention in humans is dipping by the day. The remote is with your audience and channel switch happens in less than five seconds!

Keep your story interesting, take tweaks to keep the curiosity on.

Avoid too many layers in your communication with excessive 'IF's and But's' or complicate it with too many characters, procedures, or Call to Actions, making it confusing for your viewer / reader to understand and give you the desired response.

*Segment III – B:*

*Self Care Series*

# A - Staying in Sync with nature

Diet fads have become a business in today's day and age. General health graph of human kind is only deteriorating by the day.

Unhealthy lifestyles, food habits and extremities in all walks of life eventually show their results.

When it comes to health and food, a big question is whom and what to believe?

Cornflakes says, "buy me, I will give you iron."

Wafers say, "eat me with your friends and you will enjoy the movie and tea party more than ever."

Nutritional bars say, "Be at your strongest with me."

So many dilemmas to our poor mind, isn't it?

At this difficult decision-making point, just remember one thing; your existence is part of nature. You as a human are part of nature, so everything you do - eat, drink, sleep, live must be in sync with nature, if it must be the best version. Especially the food bit, like it or not - food is one the most essential fuel that keeps you going. I am sure you will agree with me on this.

Today I am sharing few basics that make will a world of difference to your health graph at large. Any diet that has a name is a big blunder to adhere to.

Be it single food all-day diet, no carb diet, no fat diet, or the so-called magical powders of the world.

You cannot follow or in many cases even afford them life-long. We all know that imbalances of any sort never go a long way. Whenever there has been an imbalance, both perceived and experienced benefits from it have always been temporary.

The simple reason is because it is not sustainable as it does not constitute a balance. The hard truth is, as a human we may start or stop doing things at every age that we come to.

For example, in process of growing from an infant to a toddler, we start walking and then running. The same person becoming a senior citizen and with the process of ageing, slows the speed of walking, boils down to sitting or lying down.

But what is constant here is - we drink and eat as infants, toddlers, adults, and senior citizens. What changes is the quantity and may be items depending on our health conditions and medications all along. Meaning - eating is something we will be doing till our last breath and the rest is in variables.

Packaged and revamped foods are not human health-friendly. They only promote the food industry business. When I say packaged foods, I mean the entire family of ready to eats, ready to cook, just two-minute strategy and tetra packs.

I also mean all the foods that make extraordinary claims of health benefits and of course the camouflaged junks.

So be Real and Not Packaged or Revamped!

Seek your nutritional needs from natural sources and not supplements unless advised otherwise by a medical expert or then your health needs you to do so. Remember supplements are consumed to fulfil or sort deficits. They are not a replacement to natural nutrition sources.

I have come across people consuming calcium supplements but milk does not constitute their diet or then Vitamin D tablets but no effort towards getting to activity or seeking sunlight.

Very few folks understand that probiotics like ghee, curd, pickles are essentials for good gut bacteria, to absorb and assemble the Vitamin D, Calcium from both, food, supplements, and natural sunlight.

It is a good idea to be mindful with a holistic preview when you decide your food sources and choices if you desire a sustainable health graph.

Also, it is crucial to understand your very own digestive health to know which food benefits maximum and at what part of the day.

When is it most friendly to your digestion?

Did you know? Fruits and Vegetables take three hours to digest–one hour in your stomach, one hour in your small intestine, and one hour in your large intestine, while whole grains like rice and wheat need six hours each.

That is exactly why it is important to consume each of these equally crucial items in proportions and portions at suitable times of the day depending on the most active to most inactive phase of your day.

Without getting stressed or fussy with your meal plans, use this phenomenon to align with clean eating.

Foods that can give life to themselves can give life to you. For instance, if you drop some seeds of an apple into the soil, with water and sunlight, its capable of developing in to an apple tree. So, your fruits, vegetables, grains, and such whole foods are LIVE Foods because they give life.

On the other hand, if you were to burry a packet of cookies in to the soil and water it, no new cookies are going to come to life. Now, that's DEAD Food!

A food that cannot give life to itself, cannot give life to you for sure...

Also, something that most of us know yet do not know is that our life style now days has become such that our bodies barely get a chance to heal clean.

Let me simplify. If you need to heal a pot hole which is right in the middle the road, you need to fill it up, sure. but before that you need to stop the moving traffic there for allowing the filling to settle down and firm up.

What I mean to say is align your meals in a way that you have gap if 12 to 14 hours between dinner and breakfast. No, not about intermittent fasting but about halting the moving traffic and rest your gut to clean and heal for being optimally functional.

Moral Of the Story - Human Health - Friendly Foods are the ones that:

- Are Scientifically Sensible.
- Are Balanced in Proportions and Portions.
- Are Local and Seasonal.
- Are Traditionally Time Tested.
- Supports the National Economy & Global Ecology.
- Listens to Your Gut.

Also, we need to understand that human body architecture has been originally made for movement. So, exercise is not about what we ate yesterday. It is about celebrating what we are today.

It is about celebrating our ability to move our body's pain free, the way we desire.

Finally, when mother nature gave us our body, it was clean and clear. It is her property with us and some day we will be giving it back to Mother Nature.

Having said that, it is our responsibility to maintain it with utmost care and so we are able to do the return intact.

# B - Art of Mind Cleansing

To taste fresh new flavours of life, I first need to free my taste buds from the existing ones. Journaling is one of the most effective ways of doing this. It gives you clarity on the carry forward instances of the day, ways to close them at the earliest and set your mind free from baggage. You will learn from the day you have lived and will be able to organize your thoughts in a better way.

To keep yourself free from the unrequired dramas of the day, spare 10 minutes before bedtime to write your day. Good - Bad - Ugly, pen it down.

Do not try to create a flow, just write as it comes to your mind. Get it off your system. Once you finish, read what you have written as a third person.

Trust me, a lot of realizations will come by you about your thoughts and actions, how required or not they were, what were the possible alternatives you could have looked at, how you could have handled the situations differently and lots more.

You as a third person reading your day journal will also realize what about someone else's thoughts or actions disturbed or troubled you during the day and what should your approach to it be.

Sharing my personal experience, I have been journaling for quite some time now. It has helped me big time. It taught me the difference between living my journey and assuming that I am living my journey while I am not.

When we peep into ourselves, evaluate what we are going to do or what and how we want to do - things and action it out, we are living our journey but when we look at what people are doing or think of what and how they should have done or should do a thing, we are living their life.

The truth is we exist in this world to live our journey. We can live, should and do live parallel journeys with our dear ones, and probably share our journeys with them and vice versa but for sure cannot and should not live their journey.

So, a question here is why?

If I love the ones close to me, why can't I live at least some part of their journey - is thinking about them wrong?

Am I supposed to be so selfish?

No, it is not. Thinking about someone close to your heart is obvious.

Even I do. It could be right from a parent to a sibling, mentor, best friend, or spouse, would - be to even someone I am just getting to know. I may not be able to tell that specific person as to how important he or she is to me, which does happen at times. But my daily routine does include praying for that person.

When I have conversations with my people, sure we share our experiences, do a lot of listening as well, suggest stuff to each other, laugh, cry - everything, for that matter, I tell them that I love them.

All of this is real and fine, but what is incorrect is - within your mind, going on to analysing what and why people are doing, how they should be doing it, or why they are doing or not doing something or they should be doing things by your perspective to it or then discussing them with yourself or other people is getting in to their piece of the world, which is disrespectful towards someone you claim you love or even for a normal acquaintance that matters in your life.

It is only right to maintain the sanctity of a person's privacy and space to live. Besides, growth is something everyone wants and talks about.

Self-growth is the most integral part of growth. It is an inwards phenomenon and not outwards. Inward here means your journey and outward - someone else.

Journaling is not only an effective mind cleanser, but it also eventually helps you find your core.

# C - **Upgrading Your Sub-Conscious**

We all go through lots each day without even realising that we do. In our work space, with family, with friends, with our partner, with our children, with ourselves, with almost every equation of our life. Unknowingly many of us, create pile up deep within especially if what we have gone through is hurtful. For instance, some disbelief, awkward statement, or behaviour or then an uncalled-for change.

We may say whatever but change is something not easily digestible by many. It is a different story that one must eventually accept and move on for self-harmony. Though the hard truth is that the only thing that is 'consistent' and 'constant' in our life is change.

To be in harmony with change, Upgrade is unavoidable. Upgrade our subconscious, so we do not end up reminding ourselves of things that we have somewhere accepted and taken along. We do not end up with a discomfort in the subconscious or unknowingly end up scratching wounds that are in the process of healing or have just healed.

Most importantly we do not end up publicizing our delicate threads at incorrect places or to irrelevant people because that is of no help to any one, anyways.

Now that we know, upgrading our subconscious is so very crucial, how to we practice it in a few simple steps.

Let me share how I do it:
- Understand there is a change.
- Understand why you need to accommodate the change.
- Accept there is a change.
- Accept the change itself.
- Meditate the change.
- Practice the change.

Easier said than done, I know. But it is not impossible either...

## D - The 4 R Tool

Human life has complexities beyond imagination. Actively or passively these complexities do create disturbances in our inner and outer environments.

The 4R Technique has helped me big time whenever I have needed to fix any of these threads.

Here is an attempt to share the 4R Tool:

Once you have identified what is to be fixed, let us get to the 1st R:

### R – Removal

Just like it takes 21 days to form a habit, it takes the same time to remove anything that exist in your environment and is untoward. For instance, if you are having gut issues, remove the foods that are not that are not gut friendly.

If your friend or a close nit is causing you discomfort and refuses to realize it, remove from her or him the power to affect you temporarily, aiding you to heal, not removing your connection or friendship of course.

### The 2nd R is: R- Replacement

Now that you have removed the foods causing trouble to your gut, figure out how to replace them with alternatives. Of course, there will be a lot of things at the Removal stage that you just cannot replace overnight especially when it comes to relationships. For a fact, people you love the most tend to hurt you the most and then behave as though nothing ever happened. The harder truth is that you cannot change what is outside but what you can do something about is what is within.

There may be a bit of a wait-watch element here till you reach the 3rd R.

Sometimes a detached approach element helps gain perspective.

The 2nd R tool works well with handling toxicity though. Replacement gives us

- The strength to Withhold and Absorb.
- The strength to speak up at the right time and the right place with the right set of people, to recognise these before you share.
- The strength to keep yourself in the centre and at the peripherals.
- The strength to accept that your emotions to your attachments are beautiful, they are your own. No one and just no one has the right to mess around with them.

### The 3rd R is: R - Repair

This R is to work on the damage and minimize its effect.

With your health, obtain the necessary professional help based on requirements. Practice the replacements incorporated.

With people, we strengthen ourselves from within once we have withdrawn the power of giving us discomfort from that equation.

Seek to give out instances to test the waters and check if there is any trace of change. Take this phase to give yourself enough space to decide.

With situations and mindsets, plan out your actionable.

### The final - fourth R is: R - Reinforce

The first and second R also gives us a hidden power i.e. the strength to keep in our environment the 3/4th of the glass that was full while we attempt to fix the 1/4th of the empty glass.

Reinforcing is about focusing on what is there, building on it and building on what we have added or decided. This phase may also tell us to ignore the 1/4th part of the glass that is empty!

# E - Freedom within or without boundaries?

Hey, remember the famous scrabble game we played as children? I think that was one of the most out-of-the-box metrics to enhance vocabulary! Freedom means different to different people and professions.

To me, it means, the journey of 'nowhere' to 'now here'.

Let us dive into the inner artist and set you free! No matter what you do, whether you are a student, a teacher, or a chef, you have a hidden instinct that allows you a full breath.

You know, I never thought I would be into gardening, but after watching a few YouTube tutorials, I decided to give it a try. Now, I am growing a mini flower garden!

Pro tip 1: Stay Curious - Keep your eyes wide open and your mind ready to explore. Every day is a new adventure, so why not embrace it? Try something new, trying a quirky recipe. You never know where inspiration might strike!

I never realized how much writing had in common with me until I started reading and experimenting with my articulations. Now, I have my own a BlogSpot with more than 70 pieces authored by me.

Pro tip 2: Connect the Dots-Look for patterns and connections in the world around you. Sometimes, the most amazing people and thought lines come from putting pieces of your inner being together. That is exactly what Dr. Swati Lodha did to me!

I had this crazy idea for a story where a banana, was the main lead and instead of brushing it off, I decided to run with it. Now, I am helping a friend with her children's book!

Pro tip 3: Follow Your Gut-Trust your instincts and wear your emotions with pride. They are yours. Do not be afraid to jot down your thoughts, so far as they do not trouble. They not only bring you an equilibrium but often turn into something incredible!

I used to have a messy workspace cluttered with old papers and random knick-knacks. But once I cleaned it up and organized everything, I found myself feeling more focused than ever before!

Pro tip 4: Clear the Clutter-Get rid of anything that is holding you back from your being. Whether it is de-cluttering your desk or simplifying your schedule, a little tidying up can go a long way.

I never thought I would end up volunteering at a local NGO, but when a friend invited me to join them one day, I decided to give it a shot. Now, I am having the time of my life playing with little children and giggling like a child myself!

Pro tip 5: Embrace the Unknown-It is tough and I am still learning parts of it. But it is a good idea to learn from uncertainty and welcome the unexpected with open arms.

Finally, either you win or you learn, so there is very little to lose!

After all, your life is your canvas, so paint it with your uniqueness!

# F - Early Bird Realizations

An author, who is the head nurse of a hospital in Australia was on duty, looking after patients who were on their death beds. Through her journey. she has interacted with more than ten thousand dying patients, due to age and illness both. Through her conversations with her patients, she realised that though there were no similarities in them but most of the dying patients had similar regrets.

In her book, the author has shared the 'Top Five Regrets' dying patients have.

Let us take our learning's from this to stay in the best versions... while we breathe and beyond.

Regret No 1: I wish I had lived my life the way I wanted to and not got bogged down with what others think feel or say.

This is not about being a rebel. It is about taking a stand for what you believe in while you maintain the sanctity of your environment.

Regret No 2: I wish I had not been a pure workaholic. This no-where means you do not work towards achieving your professional goals. But if you are doing it at the cost of your health or loved ones. It is time to re-think. If this minute going by is not going to come back, you are paying a phenomenally heavy price for your definition of success.

Make time for your loved ones and for people who love you even if both are not the same. Most of the times, both will not be the same!

Once gone, it is a no return formula.

Regret No 3: I wish I would have been able to express what I felt.

Well, I know that is a tough call because not everyone understands it.

But do make sure you confess the due love, care, hurt and apology towards concerned people. Just remember, it is a big-time self-help tool. Use it.

Regret No 4: I wish I could have stayed connected to my people.

Like I said earlier, once gone, it is a no return formula.

Regret No 5: I wish I would have let myself stay happy.

We all know what makes us smile and gives us a space of peacefulness. Please do not let-go of it!

## G - Reflections, my piece of life...

Three hundred and sixty-five days, slide out from a tightly closed fist just like sand and wind, year after year. What went right? What did I learn? On the conclusion, I am sharing my piece of life with you....

- Life is all about Metamorphosis - Change is the only constant and consistent element of life.
- Accepting the unexpected is maturity - This is what it is. Accept what is.
- Allow yourself to heal - Forgive and forget. If you can do both, manage one at least.
- Beauty lies in connection - Connect to the universe.
- Let go of perfection - Focus on progress because that is what matters.
- Freedom within and without boundaries - Strike a balance.
- People will see only what you show - Make informed choices.
- People and situations will come and go but you will need you. Self-care is top on priority.
- Trust your inner voice - Believe in yourself.
- Subscribe to Self-Development - Your inner journey is your own.

I would love to hear from you on
**aditi.gosalia@gmail.com**
Connect with me on:
**https://www.linkedin.com/in/aditigosalia**

Until we meet with the next....

## *About the Author:*

A beacon of empowerment in the realm of education and mentorship, Aditi Gosalia carries with her over a decade of enriching experience in education management and has passionately guided thousands of learners across diverse disciplines from management to media, students to professionals instilling essential life skills and fostering career progression. Aditi's journey, marked by roles across organizations like MET League of Colleges, CMS, NIIT and Boston Computers across the last decade and a half coupled with her educational qualifications in Human Resources, Business Management, Training, Educational Leadership, Health, and Wellness exemplifies a commitment to holistic education and professional development. She is currently with Podar World College, Podar Education Network where in, she bridges academia with corporate realms, shaping futures and nurturing talent. Beyond her illustrious career, Aditi is a certified practicing life coach, dedicated to aiding others in navigating life's challenges with resilience and purpose. Her impact extends globally, as she has been recognized with accolades including 'Excellence in Professional Mentorship' and also been acclaimed as an 'Influential Leader in Soft Skills and Life Skills'.

# Reader's Notes:

www.ingramcontent.com/pod-product-compliance
Lightning Source LLC
LaVergne TN
LVHW061550070526
838199LV00077B/6983